Dance Therapy

Dance Therapy

Narrative case histories of therapy sessions with six patients

Helene Lefco

Nelson-Hall nh **Chicago**

ISBN 0–911012–93–1

Library of Congress Catalog Card Number: 73–88511

For information address
Nelson–Hall Company, Publishers,
325 W. Jackson Blvd., Chicago, Ill. 60606

Manufactured in the United States of America

To Naomi Dank; hospital administrator, editorial
consultant, friend—this book could not have been written
without her insistence and persistence.

Contents

Nothing so clearly and inevitably reveals the inner man than movement and gesture. It is quite possible if one chooses to conceal and dissimulate behind words or paintings or statues, or other forms of human expression, but the moment you move, you stand revealed, for good or evil for what you are.

—Doris Humphrey, as quoted in *The Dance Has Many Faces*, edited by Walter Sorell

Dance Therapy

Introduction

Although many books, papers, and monographs have been written on dance therapy, nowhere is there a book that tells a budding dance therapist in simple terms how to walk into a room where ten psychotic patients are waiting, how to face them, and how to help them.

This book is addressed to doctors, nurses, ancillary therapists, students, relatives and friends of the patients, and to anyone who would like to learn about the therapeutic technique of dance therapy.

What *is* dance therapy?

Dance therapy is an art and a skill which relies upon man's basic urge to dance. When professionally practiced, it illuminates for the patient the importance of the fusion of mind and body. Dance therapy promotes an integration which is necessary for psychic and physical well-being.

Dance and dance therapy must not be confused. Dance is a well-defined, structured pattern of movement that is balanced and contained. Dance therapy, on the other hand, does not deal with balanced or contained patterns, nor does it utilize the art of the performing dancer. Rather, dance therapy exists in a maelstrom of human abandonment, with the dance therapist pitting her skills against the dehumanizing effects of neurosis, psychosis, alcoholism, drug addiction, autism, and a host of behavioral problems that may affect the patient.

The task of the dance therapist is to encourage a patient to move his body. To do this, the therapist borrows from the crafts of the calisthenics teacher, the dancer, and the psychiatrist. A trained therapist is unburdened by a morass of procedures and is free to initiate and discard in order to find the most potent tool to aid in effecting the union of mind and body. Ultimately, through the release of dance and through the therapist's observations, the patient may gain an awareness of self and an understanding of the part that emotions play in the stance, form, and movement of his body.

There is no standard dance form for dance therapy. Any dance that appeals to the patient may be used. Primitive dance, African tribal dance, folk dance, the waltz, the polka, and even rock can be used effectively. Interpretive movement, the dance "miming" of music by the patient, a technique perfected to an art form by Isodora Duncan, also can be of great therapeutic value to the patient.

The dance therapist is primarily, but not exclusively, a dancer, conscious of her own body and its functioning. Since a dancer's body is her instrument, she, more than any other person, is aware of the importance of bodily health, vitality, and adaptability. Though technique, theory, improvisation, and choreography are primarily skills of the dancer, they may be used to great advantage by the dance therapist. However, a dance therapist must discard the more disciplined techniques of a dancer, leaving specific rules of expertise to the concert stage.

Even more important than dance training is the personality of the dance therapist. She should be sufficiently aware of other persons so that she is able to respond quickly to nonverbal cues. She must be able to remain optimistic in a deeply troubled atmosphere, for aside from her proficiency, it is her spirit and wit and heart that will enable her to lift the gloom at the start of each session.

I have studied the disciplines of Graham, Holm, Wigman, Weidman, Humphrey, and Limón. I learned the basics of dance therapy by studying with therapists in New York, Philadelphia, and Washington, D.C., and by working as a dance therapist, first at a state hospital with regressed, tranquilized cases, then later at a private hospital with unmedicated patients. I had the good fortune to participate in a series of training sessions with the pioneer dance therapist, Marian Chace, whose influence upon me, both personally and professionally, has been profound. A truly sensitive and intuitive woman who came to each session with astounding freshness and flexibility, Marian Chace taught me by example that a dance therapist's greatest asset is an instinctive joy in movement. It is this primal spontaneity which must be transmitted to her patients.

For those dance-oriented people who would like to become dance therapists, there are many courses and programs available for the undergraduate and graduate college student. (More specific information on requirements for dance therapy certification is listed in Chapter Nine.)

*   *   *

This book is about my dance therapy sessions with Carol, Penny, Brian, Kevin, Don, and Laura. Since quick results with patients are rare—there is a ritualistic time for them to show you their wares, while they check to see what *you* are selling —I have tried to dramatize in my chapters only those moments which signal behavioral changes.

The reader will note that I am rarely addressed the same way twice by my patients. I was called only "Mrs. Lefco" in the formal atmosphere of the state hospital, where I first worked and where the line between patient and therapist was clearly defined. At the clinic, the setting for this book, there was less distinction between people, less barriers, less formality. I began as "Mrs. Lefco" and quickly switched to "Helene." Today, I am called almost everything, including, "Hey, you, crazy person!" The dance therapist answers to many names—and to anyone who calls.

Although I generally have as many as twelve patients in a session, I have concentrated only on the six who were long-term inpatients at the private clinic where I worked. The shortest amount of time I spent with a patient was one year; the longest was five years. The names used are fictitious, but there is no fiction in my recounting of those special moments when all guards were down, when my patients chose to cast off their armor and trust me. Those moments were very real.

From such moments and from such trust come the miracle of change.

4

CHAPTER I

The Group

"If I were wearing my high-heeled, pointy shoes I'd ram 'em up your ass—three inches—till they came out your tonsils! You creep!," shouted Carol, propelling a stream of spit that landed squarely in my eye.

I knew of no reason for Carol's hostility toward me, so I could only assume that this young woman's anger was actually directed toward something or someone, perhaps even toward herself. Whatever the target, she had not been able to release her fury, until I floated innocently into her ken, becoming "it"—the recipient of her pent-up rage. Judging from her dilated pupils, her ramrod-stiff body, and the pallor of her face, I knew immediately that Carol meant business.

I also knew that a direct confrontation on my part might lead Carol into screaming resistance or into the full-scale violence of a physical encounter. Looking again into Carol's face,

I decided to leave the technique of confrontation to her psychiatrist. As a dance therapist, I thought it best to encourage Carol to release her anger by using a *symbolic* punching bag, and not me.

Carol continued to glare at me, and when I made no immediate response, she gestured obscenely in my direction. I was actually relieved to see her use a gesture which, compared to her former, threatening belligerence, seemed quite harmless. Breathing hard with anxiety, I marched quickly over to the record player and put on an African record that I knew Carol loved: Fela Ransome-Kuti and the Africa '70, an album full of the sound of trumpets, saxophones, and drums.

Standing at a safe distance from Carol, I stamped my feet and crouched my body in an African war dance position. Carol stood quietly at the other end of the room, watching me. I was aware that she might simply snatch the record from the record player and smash it on the floor. But from beneath Carol's tight jeans, I suddenly spotted motion, slight and tentative. As her knees bent, I knew that some tension was leaving her legs. Then, almost in spite of herself, Carol's body let loose in a spontaneous explosion of primitive passion. She slammed her feet hard against the concrete floor, crumpled her torso, and let her head with its long hair whip forward and back. She pummeled the air with her fists and let out a cry that sounded like the coloratura shriek of an exotic bird's mating call. Carol danced to the end of the cut, and then, perspiring and spent, fell into a chair. She threw back her head and closed her eyes, her violence spent.

That incident happened last week. Today, on my way to the clinic, an hour's trip that takes me through the city's heavily trafficked streets into winding stretches of country lanes, I wonder what will await me as I once again set foot in the recreation room. Not that anything can scare me off, for the clinic where I work has an oddly seductive power over me. Offers from more conveniently located hospitals come and go, but still I stay committed to this highly controversial mental hospital tucked away in the rolling hills of Pennsylvania.

The clinic is a sprawling compound, not physically attractive and more gypsy encampment than mental hospital. Mobile trailers dot the fourteen-acre piece of farmland. Brought in for some forgotten purpose, the trailers have sprouted roots in the rich country soil and now house the clinic's autonomous units of patients and therapists. The grounds are erratically planted and cared for. Flowers and bushes, once tended when a patient's mood was high, either spring up through the grass, or lie choked by weeds in a conventional flower bed. Horticulturally, this place is a far cry from the usual mental hospital where trees were diligently labeled and orderly concrete paths lead to the familiar comfort of a park bench and potted geraniums.

These agrarian symbols of free, personal expression are the visitor's first clue to the treatment given here, for the clinic's focus is overwhelmingly on the patients. For some of the patients, this is the first time they have been permitted to live in an atmosphere free of destructive criticism. For others, it is their initial attempt to turn their backs on obsessive neatness and perfectionism. Parents and families may look askance at the patients' work—unfinished gardens and misspelled signs abound on the property—but, here again, it is the patients' work and the patients' needs rather than the standards of the visitor that shape the policy of the clinic.

Perhaps my experience as a dance therapist at a state hospital has made me a strong proponent of this type of natural environment, "milieu" therapy, for I have seen the empty faces and the devitalized bodies of patients housed and cared for in large, orderly, antiseptically clean buildings. There they sit, stupified, behind whitewashed walls and three sets of locked doors, in an atmosphere of pessimism and indifference. How many light-years away is this from the kind of good-humored, optimistic, twenty-four-hours-a-day therapy that is practiced at the clinic?

Here, three to five patients and two staff therapists live in trailers or in cottages located on the acreage. In these "households," a family setting is approximated in the hope that the patient will relearn emotional reactions and interpersonal relationships. Participation in all facets of family life, from shared work responsibilities to leisure activities, such as trips, swimming, games, cookouts, and parties, are constantly interspersed with therapy from various staff members.

At the physical center of the clinic lies an Early American-style farmhouse building, which contains the staff offices. Behind this is the red barn, the focus of all recreational activities, including dance therapy, art therapy, and music therapy.

Dogs, cats, rabbits, and basketballs are an integral part of life on this tract of land. The patients, here, because of the clinic's policy, are very different souls from the tranquilized robots living in the state hospitals. Drugs are given to those patients whose violent drives may cause them to harm themselves or others. For the most part, however, patients here are left undrugged and free to suffer. There is no attempt to ameliorate their symptoms; instead, patients are allowed to respond to their problems in a sympathetic atmosphere.

As a dance therapist, I find these patients exciting to work with. They may resist me, they may insult me, they may "con" me, or even call me a string of four-letter words—and they might even like me! Whatever their behavior, it is responsive and gives me an opportunity to channel their release of emotion into body movement.

Today, as I turn into the clinic's driveway, I spot teen-aged Kevin loping toward my car. For the past six months he has faithfully waited for my car to arrive so that he could offer to help me carry the records. Although it is difficult to understand his "word-salad" mumbling, Kevin's generous intent is obvious to me. It is particularly touching in a boy who four years ago was given up by his parents as a social menace. I never refuse Kevin his request, although sometimes in the excitement of the moment he may drop the records or stumble off with them in the wrong direction. But there is charm and softness in this tall, gangling boy who once almost killed his brother with a golf club.

Seventeen-year-old Laura, five-feet tall and weighing over two hundred pounds, is standing just inside the barn door. Her slack brown hair hangs over her sallow face; her arms seem to be pasted to the side of her gargantuan body. When she sees me, there is the trace of a smile around the edges of her mouth. Wordlessly, she follows me. Once inside, with Kevin shuffling close beside me, his hand making little staccato pats on my shoulder, with Laura, heavy and silent in my wake, I assess the condition of my other patients.

Don is sitting quietly on the couch, his head in his hands. At twenty-four, Don is a pale, blond, tentative man, who seems to be trying to withdraw from the brute contact of the world of men. Brian is pacing restlessly around the room. A former prep school and college hero with a drug-infested past, Brian is now thirty-five, and is, in a sense, the hardest patient for me to reach. Being older than the others, he has been away from reality for the longest time. He is removed, convoluted, arch. He has a brilliant mind, manifested by his facility with language, his metaphors, his philosophic bent. Penny is lying on her back on the couch, biting her lower lip, her young forehead creased with lines of anxiety. The baby of the group, Penny is fourteen. She is a tense, angry, beautiful girl who lacks assurance of her beauty. She is beginning to accept the fact that she must drop her enormous defenses in order to lessen, maybe even cure, her epileptic seizures. Carol is sitting cross-legged on the floor smoking a cigarette, fingering her long necklace with nervous tugs. At twenty, she is a desperately empty, seeking girl, almost a burnt-out case. She hopes that the clinic will show her how to approximate the satisfactions that she once knew in a drug culture.

What has brought these desperate people to a mental hospital? These patients have no "labels," for the clinic feels that once a patient is labeled, not only the therapist, but also the patient, has to confirm the diagnosis, and the kind of flexibility of treatment that the clinic proffers is summarily blocked. One thing is certain: These inpatients are here because for the most part, they are delicate, vulnerable, retreated figures who, for one reason or another, have slipped away from reality. They have come here via different routes: heroin addiction, criminal behavior, sexual promiscuity, victims of too many acid trips, and severe cases of alcoholism, as well as knife-wielding, bat-swinging behavioral problems.

The room in the barn where I work is a large, friendly arena, decorated in the slaphappy style that is characteristic of the clinic, not really spotless and certainly not orderly. Nonetheless, this room suits us. It is not too modern, not too clinical, not too big. It has a homey quality.

On the walls hang the patients' art work: a few headless, eviscerated bodies in pastels, as well as some crayon drawings of fragmented heads and legs and arms; an oil painting showing a huge tree; a dark, foreboding, windowless house with a tiny black door made fast by a huge lock. In a corner stands a large paper mâché Santa Claus with breasts, known to everyone as "Mrs. Santa." There is a set of drums, a few resident kittens, a ping-pong table at one end, and a pool table at the other. A pillow, torn apart by some patient's rage, lies on the floor, its stuffing strewn about. We have a hard-surfaced area for dancing, a small, carpeted section for floor work, a couch, and some comfortable chairs for the listening and reflection that sometimes conclude the session.

Laura, obese, listless, feet dragging, pants hanging, taps my forearm.

"You gonna dance?" she asks.

"You bet," I say.

Quickly, I set up my record player and pull off my shoes. On an impulse, I put on a Strauss waltz. I find that the kids have an automatic physical response to rock, (which they love), so that an unfamiliar musical beat, like the waltz, calls upon their creativity. I spread my arms wide, beginning to sway with the three-quarter rhythm.

"Anybody for a waltz?" I ask, half-dancing around the room.

It is a curious phenomenon, but since I expect the patients to dance, they do. Maybe not everyone at once, but there is never a time that at least one or two patients do not

11

rise to the occasion, with the music and the dance therapist providing encouragement. The patients may look like the walking wounded as they shuffle out to the center of the room, but they come.

Many times, Penny, her delicate young figure curled womblike on the couch, will present me with an hour's worth of resistance. Or possibly Don will stand with his back to the group, his blond hair falling over his face, his muscles taut with hostility, his body unyielding. Just having him turn around to face the group might take the length of the session, if I'm lucky. But the remarkable fact is that eventually Penny and Don *do* join the group.

I am elated to have a good response today.

"Hey kids, let's form a circle," I say over the music. "Everybody grab a hand!"

I am certain that it astounds the patients that, in spite of furious faces and impassive bodies and negative stances, a circle is formed. As often as it happens, even I am impressed by this phenomenon. Hands interlock in the impersonal safety of a circle, hands which minutes before would have tolerated no human touch. Bodies press together. There is an audible sigh from Don. Penny's shoulders, habitually hunched protectively around her neck, now drop their guard. A delighted smile lights Kevin's face.

My plan is to have no plan for each session so that the patients can be free to express their emotions in impulsive movement. A lesson format with its attendant expectations might block the spontaneity that springs brilliantly into focus when a patient's response is uncensored and unbounded by himself—or by me.

But nonetheless, I do find that the circle is one of the

most effective formations for getting the patients to become aware of one another. Left to their own devices, the patients would respond to the music in a separate, isolated manner. And, although self-exploration is certainly encouraged, communicating through touch is an even more vital part of dance therapy. In a circle, even the most withdrawn patient is forced to acknowledge the presence of another by the subtle pressure or the tense grip of a handclasp.

As we move to the music, Carol begins to swing her arms in a soft, romantic way; quite a departure from her typical, hard-rock, aggressive style. Her chest opens to the ceiling, her throat is thrust forward, her head back. The tension in her shoulders relaxes. She waltzes like the romantic of a bygone era.

"That's lovely, Carol," I say.

Brian looks at her. "You could be a child on a spring day in the school playground."

For a moment Carol dances on, charmingly—and then, suddenly, she stops and makes a face.

"Christ, Brian, did you have to say that?"

"What did he say?" I ask.

"Ah, that bit about the school playground really pisses me off—that was a bad scene."

"Why?" I ask, my arms still swinging in three-quarter time.

Carol, beginning to waltz again, speaks softly. "Well, it's like I always had a deep voice—even then—and the bastards at the playground wouldn't play with me. They said I was a boy." Carol's arms swung up in the air, taking the arms of Laura and Don up with her. Suddenly she twists her hips and makes the swing into the slice of a karate chop.

I twist my hips and shoot my arms up, still holding fast to Brian and Penny.

"Let's give the bastards a group karate," I say.

Holding hands, we swing one another around roughly, our bodies whipping together in a strong karate movement.

Carol giggles. "Wow! This would blow the mind of one Johann Strauss!"

The pain of her past recollection aired and acted upon, Carol now feels free to waltz by herself, arms rounded, head inclined; a veritable Viennese lady. The circle dissolves naturally, as patients drop the hands they were holding.

I watch carefully as knees bend, as one solar plexus after another seems to dissolve its tension. Facial muscles, habitually downturned, change shape before my eyes, as mouths turn up into smiles. Perhaps it is the lilt of the music; perhaps it is the primitive rapture that comes from basic body movement. Whatever the reason, each time I have a dance therapy session I am impressed with the instantaneous transformation of some of the patients.

Other patients, however, fight experiencing pleasurable sensations. Today, Laura is highly resistant. She is cranky, angry, withdrawn, but is nonetheless making perfunctory motions to keep me "off her back." At present, I am satisfied with that, on the grounds that some motion for Laura is much better than her yielding to an immobilized, catatonic posture. Don is moving tenuously, in his own way, but his body is still quite tense. His neck continues to assume the typical wry twist that angles his head off from his body, as if his head were trying to avoid admitting a relationship with his body.

As the waltz plays on, I pull my neck out to one side.

"Hey, Don, what's it like to have your head out here?"

14

Don's eyes flash at me. "Good. I really dig it."

"You like to be that far from your body?" I ask.

"Don't hassle me!" he says.

I pull my head back in position. "But this way, I get a good feeling . . . like I'm putting it all together."

Don carefully moves his head into a position where it fits squarely on his neck. He laughs and looks down at his slight frame.

"OK, I've got it together now. So what's so beautiful about that?"

Kevin is watching interestedly. He walks over to Don and stares at him.

"You look cool, Don, really cool," he says, patting Don on the back with the little staccato pats he bestows on friends.

Don grins. "Thanks. It really feels crazy . . . but," Don shrugs his shoulders, "once you're into it, it's not bad."

As Kevin tries a little neck movement of his own, his large, curly head shaking back and forth, I sense that some Indian music might be more appropriate for isolated neck movements. I change the record to Ali Akbar's "Flowers of Evil," an exotic sound of sarod and lute.

Brian's ears perk up at the sound of the lute, as he locks his hands around the back of his neck and begins to move sensually. Suddenly Carol's arms fly over her head, and she begins using her neck muscles like an Indian dancer. Effortlessly, smoothly, as if a string were attached to her ears, she moves her neck muscles horizontally, her face held forward, her eyes straight ahead and shining with triumph as she moves her head from side to side.

"Wow," Penny says in awe of Carol's proficiency. "That's really groovy."

Carol grins. "You know, I could really get into this Eastern culture stuff. It's as good as grass—it really turns me on."

Now the group is following Carol's lead, as they experiment with different neck positions. Only Laura stands alone, staring up in the corner of the room.

"Laura," I call out sharply.

Laura is startled out of her reverie. She looks up at me guiltily. "This music is a drag," she says.

"OK, Laura," I say. "How about putting on some music that you like?"

Laura walks slowly to the record player. Though she rummages through the stack of records, she can't find one she likes. The sound of the sitar continues to fill the room.

Carol is still performing, and as Don watches he attempts to move his neck around. For a moment his neck is perfectly aligned. He smiles as he feels the difference between his former head position and the new one.

Fourteen-year-old Penny, looking relaxed and calm, now nods her head to the music. At this moment she has the serenity of an Indian guru, and it is difficult to imagine the passion she experienced a year ago, when she had tried to kill herself with a bread knife.

As Penny nods, so do I, enlarging her nod, making it grow more affirmative. Penny, a quick study, begins to permit her whole body to act out the idea of "yes."

"Yes!" says Penny's head, neck, eyes, chin, mouth. Her feet stomp assertively. There is no mistaking the power of her affirmation. I stomp along with Penny, empathizing, mirroring, as I move toward the record player. Quickly, I switch to some contemporary rock, "Santana," where the drum beat will match the strong, steady motions I am seeing.

"Yes! Yes!" I shout, as I once again join Penny. The other patients are involved now, taking up the cry. Stomping and shouting, the group lifts their knees high off the floor, letting their feet come down hard, forcing them into a kind of reality base-touching, something the three men patients need particularly.

"Yes, you bet your ass!" Don says softly, but not so quietly that anyone misses it. I look up in time to see him smile with great satisfaction.

"My mother always says that," he adds; his way of covering himself for any emotional outburst that makes him feel like a man.

The group has been titillated by Don's phrase. "You bet your ass! You bet your ass!" they chant. Don's smile gives way to a deep rumble that in turn loosens up into a belly laugh for all of us.

I begin to notice some animation in Laura. For most of the session she has stood truculently by the record player, her body stiff, her face set in hard lines. Now the dull look has left her green eyes and she seems sharper. The patients around me are momentarily all of a piece, jolly and affirmative. Laura, whose first response to everything was "no," seems now to be shaking her head negatively, her straight, lank hair covering her face with each sidewise movement.

"Laura," I call, "that's good. C'mon over here so we can follow what you're doing."

Laura's "no" now has the proper impetus. Of course, she won't come over to us. All two hundred pounds of her is saying "no" with undeniable force. She is a Mt. Rushmore of negativism, as she grits her teeth, plants her feet on the ground, and angles her elbows into her broad waist in one mountainously negative gesture.

All of us drift toward Laura. Her "no" is catching on fast. There is a great amount of "no" present in the room. In a moment, fists are clenched, light punches are traded, and assaultive anger seems to be lurking in each patient's eyes. Brian grabs my shoulder as we push first playfully, then forcefully, against one another. I feel his fingers gripping my shoulders.

It is ineffective, even dangerous, for a dance therapist to confront an assaultive patient with her own fearful response. Aside from the physical injury she might receive, forceful confrontation is not what the patient needs from her. The patient is begging to win a psychic battle. An inventive dance therapist might change an assaultive movement into a dance by using the leverage of a striking arm as the fulcrum in a push-pull mock battle. In this case, gauging Brian's aggression, I decided not to risk any physical encounter.

Quickly, I sink to the floor at Brian's feet.

"You've got me, Brian," I say, hanging my head.

It takes a few seconds for Brian's iron grip on my shoulders to relax. Then he smiles down at me, the gallant winner. With a supportive hand, he helps me up. Our fingers entwine, but for only a moment.

Because I am breathing hard and feeling the effects of our session, I am certain that the time has come for the patients to relax as well. We all sit down on the carpet in a circle, feet touching, arms around each other. We close our eyes and let James Taylor's "Sweet Baby James" wash over us. Then we do yoga deep breathing. I do the slow counts as I watch stomachs rise and fall at a slow, even tempo.

I look around at my patients as they sway comfortably against one another and shake my head when I recall what they looked like two hours ago. Without any preconceived plan, the session has been packed full of emotions freely and spontaneously expressed. The patients have even experienced a basic principle of therapy, "If a person cannot say 'no,' his 'yes' is meaningless." (Alexander Lowen, *The Body in Therapy* [New York: Macmillan and Co., 1967]).

My eyes travel to Laura, to her shining face, flushed and alive. I look around at the others—Brian, Kevin, Penny, Don, and Carol—and hope that their day will be happier for having had this dance therapy session.

CHAPTER II

The Rich Girl Who Stole Food

LAURA

I walked into the recreation room a half hour in advance of my dance therapy session, a usual practice that allowed me time to set up my record player, choose my records, sweep up cigarette butts, and cajole the clinic cats into prowling elsewhere. Standing just inside the door, her face blank, her eyes focused on the ceiling, was my young patient, Laura. I was not surprised to see her, for she frequently arrived early for some one-to-one attention. However, today I was shocked to see Laura wearing a large, cardboard sign around her neck, which read, "I steal food from children."

"Hi, Laura," I said. "What's that all about?"

Laura kept her eyes on the ceiling, a small smile playing around her mouth.

"Laura! Laura! Laura!" I called with increasing volume. My experience with hallucinating patients made me fairly certain that Laura was in fact responding to her voices. The focus of her eyes and her secret smile were my clues.

"Laura!" I shouted.

Finally, Laura's pale-green eyes adjusted to my presence. She pointed to the sign around her neck. "They wanted you to see this," she said.

Laura stood in front of me stolidly, her massive two-hundred-pound frame giving her a five-by-five appearance. Though only seventeen, she looked about thirty years old. Her body was poker stiff, her legs pillars of rounded fat that seemed to meld into an impenetrable mass. She stared vacantly at me.

"What's it mean?" I asked.

"Can't you read, dummy?"

"Yes, Laura," I said, ignoring the jibe and the hostility. "It says that you steal food from children. Is that true?"

Laura's eyes focused on a space above her head, and she began to laugh uproariously.

I grasped her shoulders with my hands. "Laura," I said sharply, "listen to me! Is it true that you stole food?"

Dazedly, Laura turned to me and nodded. I knew it must have given her great pain to have to appear before me wearing that ignominious sign, for we had just begun to build a relationship based on some dancing, some talking, and a great deal of touching. But though I was filled with a sudden fury and indignation toward the family therapists for making Laura go through the anguish of this punishment, I understood that they were fighting for Laura's mental health. If shame could bring her into contact with reality, then Laura's embarrassment was actually constructive, and my indignation unimportant.

22

"Laura," I asked, tipping her several chins up toward me, "is it true that you steal food from children?"

Laura averted her eyes and brushed my hand away. "Yeah, it's true. So what? I took an apple and a lollypop from Ricky. Big deal!"

"You mean Ricky, your therapist's little boy? You stole from him?"

"Why the hell not?" Laura said. "That little squirt's allowed to go into the refrigerator—and I ain't."

Maybe the therapists were on the right track. Certainly, this explosive outburst was better than the usual unresponsive grunts that emanated from the girl who arrived six months ago with a transistor radio stuck to her ear, who used towels instead of toilet tissue, and who gave no sign that she was aware of other human beings.

"You have a little brother, don't you, Laura?" I asked.

Laura turned her back on me then and walked stiffly toward the center of the room. I had struck a nerve.

"Don't you ever shut up?" she asked over her shoulder.

I chuckled. "You know you're right, Laura. It's time for me to shut up and for us to dance."

Laura had reminded me that I was a dance therapist, a person skilled at bringing forth an emotional release through dance. Once I permitted myself to become engaged in verbal techniques, I was in a sense robbing the patient of a chance to reveal her problems through the channels of movement.

Now it was important for me to take my psychic cues from Laura and to translate them quickly into movement. Perhaps we could bring to the surface Laura's feelings toward her little brother.

I walked over to Laura, extending my arms toward her.

"OK, Laura, I've read the sign. I'm sorry it happened. Now, how about taking it off so we can dance?"

Laura's face was impassive.

I lifted the loathsome sign from her neck, putting it out of sight on a chair in the corner. "You'll probably have to wear it back to the unit after our session, but I don't think you can do much moving in here with it on."

Laura's eyes followed me as I discarded the sign. "I'll twist if you wanna," she said, flashing me a phony smile as she wheedled for food. "Got a Lifesaver or somethin'?"

Her comment suddenly made me wonder if, in fact, Laura and I had a trusting relationship, or whether she merely manipulated me in order to get candy. During Laura's first few months at the clinic, I did openly bribe her for movement with a mint or two, but clinic policy on that score was now firm: Laura was to have no food reward from any staff member.

"You know the rule, Laura," I said. "I can't give you any candy in here. But I'd love to twist. I've got a good record for you."

"Not even a stick of gum, Mrs. Lefco?"

I shook my head firmly and hurried over to the record player. Soon the blast of an old Chubby Checkers' record filled the room. I moved toward Laura, twisting my hips to the beat. How odd that she had chosen this music, when undoubtedly, she, like the rest of her generation, had been weaned on the Beatles and the Rolling Stones. The twist went back to Laura's childhood, when her mother was a young married woman. It had been that generation's first social exposure to the pelvis, and Laura's first glimpse of social dancing.

As I continued to increase the arc of my hips, I detected some movement in Laura. That great lump of a body, which for months seemed incapable of movement, now began to undulate. It wasn't a passionate action, merely an underplayed twisting of her hips, but it was movement such that the loose, flabby fat on her arms and legs began to wobble and shake. As I watched Laura, it occurred to me that it was unusual for a seventeen-year-old girl to wear clothes reminiscent of the style of the fifties. Unlike the sharp, mod outfits of her peers, Laura wore shapeless, short-sleeved, wraparound housedresses and bobby socks; outfits for Laura, which exposed vast areas of her soft, quivering flesh. Despite the expensive, fashionable costumes that her chic mother sent her through the mails, Laura clung stubbornly to her housedresses.

"You're a pretty good twister, Laura," I said.

"My mom said you should make believe you wuz drying yourself with a towel 'n then you could twist. Daddy and her did it all the time. Me and my brother usta watch."

I had a sudden vision of Laura's first week at the clinic, when she astounded her family therapists by using their clean white towels as toilet tissue. I also remembered hearing at a staff meeting discussion that Laura and her brother drank from baby bottles until they were ten years old. Their favorite drinking place had been under the couch in the living room where they had watched their young parents dance. "Twisting towels," baby bottles, a permissive, affluent mommy and daddy, sibling rivalry—what a psychiatric grab bag for Laura to choose from.

We twisted together for a few minutes, our rhythms meshing. Finally, I said to her, "Twisting can be more like

25

skiing than towel-drying, Laura. Come and ski with me."

Widening my hip movement, I beckoned to her. "C'mon, I'll race you down the mountain . . . use your hips, now . . . bend your knees, lower . . . lower . . . go much lower, Laura." As I encouraged her, Laura made a tentative attempt at allowing her massive weight to sink into her knees.

"That's it!" I called out. "You've got the idea now. Watch out for the slalom poles . . . and let's go!" Bellowing loudly, I added, "Track!"

The beat of the twist music lent itself perfectly to the race. Laura's face began to lose its stony quality, as her hips moved in a progressively wider arc.

"You've got it now, Laura," I said. "You've got the motion now. Keep it up. Keep your knees bent!"

With an impish glint in her eyes, Laura moved her tremendous girth in front of me and waggled her hips. "Hey, I'm beating you, Mrs. Lefco, but my brother, he could *really* take you!

"No, thanks, I don't need him. It looks like you're doing a good enough job on me!" I said from behind her. "But watch out! I'm breathing down your neck—here I come!"

Laura grunted with unaccustomed strain, as she artfully hopped and twisted just in front of me, successfully blocking me from passing her. But even in the heat of the race, my role as dance therapist made me aware of the deadness of Laura's arms.

"Grab your poles, Laura! You might need them for balance in those hairpin turns ahead."

Laura's chubby little arms, those two atrophied appendages, miraculously came to life, taking hold of imaginary

26

poles. Under that blubber Laura had elbows, upper arms, and strong forearms. She looked down at her arms and legs, all synchronizing beautifully, and then turned to grin triumphantly at me. Her face was crimson and perspiring from her effort. She was breathing in short spurts.

"Whaddya know? I beat you," she gasped. "Wish my brother could see me now," she said, leaning on me in exhaustion.

"What do you think he'd say?" I asked.

Laura chuckled. "That I was OK for a girl."

I put my arms around her, and Laura snuggled inside of them, catching her breath. "That male chauvinist pig's gotta go," I said.

"You can say that again!" Laura said, permitting herself to be rocked in my arms to the fast beat of the fifties. She might have enjoyed even more rocking with her dance therapist, while her thoughts, animated by the music, hovered like clouds over her childhood years. Yet, when the other patients drifted in for our session, Laura suddenly moved away from me.

"Christ!" Carol said, shaking her beautiful long hair as soon as she got an earful of the twist music. "As if I don't feel lousy enough today without listening to that vomit!"

"Oh, Carol, give us a break," I said. "Laura likes it."

"You *like* that garbage?" Carol asked incredulously. She shrugged her shoulders. "Well, what can you expect from a looney bin, anyway?" With a toss of her waist-length hair, Carol flounced off to the other end of the room.

Laura called to her. "You can change the record. I don't care. Today's a lousy day, anyway."

"Why do you say that?" I asked.

"Oh, because I didn't dance good . . . and I had to wear the sign and all. You'll probably give me a lousy grade for dancing."

"You know I don't give grades in here."

"Yeah, I know," Laura said. "You're a weirdo teacher."

I laughed. "So you think I'm a weirdo?"

Laura wiped her runny nose with the back of her hand. "Yeah, if you're supposed to be a dance teacher, how come you teach that ski crap?"

"Would you believe me if I told you that I think you did more with your body today with that 'ski crap' than you would have in the Arthur Murray studio?"

"Yeah?" Laura said. "Is that why they call this dance therapy instead of just dancing?"

"I guess you might say that," I said, "because you don't learn any steps here. You just get a feeling for what your body is saying."

"No shit? A talking body?"

"In a way, Laura," I said, "your body did talk to me today."

Laura looked down at herself. "Well, if you know so much, what is my body saying right now?"

Penny had come into the room and was standing close to Laura, listening to the conversation. "*I* know what your body's saying," said Penny, as she slipped into Laura's habitual posture, a "living comma," head down, back concave, stomach protruding. "Your body is saying, 'Look at me. I'm a fat, dead mackerel!' "

Brian walked over to us soberly and studied Penny as she mimed Laura. "It looks more like an elephant fetus to me."

"Hey, kids," Carol called from across the room, "Laura's body's clammed up on lots of stuff. Get a load of this."

Everyone turned to see Carol, who had put on Laura's sign. She was dancing around the room to Carole King's "You Make Me Feel Like a Natural Woman," simulating Laura's unique body posture.

Laura's face showed no emotion as she watched Carol's performance.

"Food. Give me food!" Carol begged. "I only weigh two hundred pounds, but I'm so hungry that I steal from babies."

I watched horrified, torn between the desire to save Laura from further hurt and the urge to help her become aware of the destructiveness of her obsession with eating.

Yet as Carol danced on, continuing her parody of Laura, the other patients hardly paid attention to her. Perhaps her mocking movements were too painful for them to stare at, or perhaps the music spoke to them on a more personal level. Carol's act finished, her audience scattered, she removed Laura's sign and sat down.

Penny, dancing in the center of the room, seemed to be preening herself, her legs spread in a confident stance, her chest thrust out, her arms held wide. Over toward the door, Kevin and Don were dancing together, tenderly looking into each other's eyes. Brian was on the small square of carpet by himself, swaying and humming to the music. Only Laura was a nonparticipant, her face a stony mask of indifference.

This seemed to be the moment for pulling all of these unrelated activities back into a cohesive group.

"Say, gang, how about forming a circle?" I suggested. "We can all be natural women, natural people, with natural appetites, like sex," and as my eyes lit on Laura's stiff body and her tense, hard face, I added, "like hunger, and stealing."

29

Laura's cheeks colored. "Don't fuck around with me, Lefco," she muttered.

Laura's allowing her anger to surface, I thought. Certainly the clinic had come down hard on her that week, hoping that she would explode in a burst of anger. For years, Laura's withdrawal into her insulating flesh had been her only defense against unbearable psychic pain. Now the clinic was intent on focusing their attack on one of Laura's problem spots—her gluttonous eating. The clinic's thinking was that although Laura could not come to grips with the whole spectrum of her traumas, she might be able to fight a small-scale war on a specific issue. Once she was battling and alive, her insights in other directions might follow.

"Wait a minute! Wait a minute!" Carol said, hopping up from her chair and dashing over to the record player. "I've got a better record for appetites. Blood, Sweat, and Tears doing 'More and More'. It's got a groovy guitar solo. But let's not do it in a circle. We need freedom for this."

Carol's musical instinct was sure. "More and More" was exactly what we needed I felt, as I watched the music and lyrics incite the patients into a grabbing kind of movement with their fingers and their arms. Soon the weight of their entire bodies seemed to be behind a snatching, taking motion. This was *not* circle time.

Don seemed especially caught up in the aggressively acquisitive movement.

"Show me how badly you want it, Don," I said.

Don responded by "taking" in a fierce way, pulling the space around him toward his body. "Yeah, I want it. It's mine," he said.

"What do you want so badly?" I asked.

30

"First place in the freestyle," he said, scooping up imaginary water with his cupped palms.

I swam freestyle alongside Don for a minute or two, a technique we had evolved together in previous dance therapy sessions. Once again we were working out the contents of Don's disturbing, recurrent dream.

"Gimme, you mothers! It's mine!" Don said belligerently, as his arms reached out in a strong Australian crawl.

We swam side by side, silently and intently, for another minute, until Kevin, sidling up to Don, took his hand and patted it.

"You're a great swimmer," he said.

Don smiled radiantly. "Thanks, kid. Thanks," he said, straightening up.

"Wanna see me do something?" Kevin asked.

Don nodded.

Kevin took a long, smooth backswing with an imaginary golf club. I shuddered as I recalled that he had almost killed a boy with a golf club when he was younger. Fortunately, this time his golf swing was nothing more than a wholesome release of energy.

"See that?" Kevin beamed. "I got it. I got my birdie."

This time it was Don who took Kevin's hand and patted it. This demonstration of their need for nonthreatening touching encouraged me to try again for a circle. Now the group came together compliantly, interested in making contact with one another. It was a warm interval of easy camaraderie, and a good break before the intensity of what I imagined would follow. Only Laura stood outside the circle, stiff and unyielding, her skin pale.

I felt Don's hand in mine tense up. He pulled himself away from the circle. "Let's do the grabbing stuff again!"

Keeping Laura in view, I asked, "Is there some food you want to grab, Don?"

Although I had chosen the topic in order to lure Laura into the circle, my suggestion seemed to generate some excitement among the other patients.

"How about some spaghetti?" Don asked, "The real garlicky, Italian stuff with lots of sauce. It really freaks me out."

"Sounds delicious," I said. "How about it, kids? Spaghetti, anyone?" I turned to Carol, who looked disapproving. "Carol, how about starting the record 'More and More' again?"

Carol shrugged, "OK, it won't make the spaghetti go down any easier, but it won't hurt either. As for me, I want some good grass!"

Don's eyes shone with excitement. Whether the idea of the slop and wetness of spaghetti and sauce intrigued him, I didn't know, but his fingers seemed almost to be caressing the imaginary spaghetti. He seemed to want to touch it, to play with it, to feel the primitive ooze of it slipping through his fingers. The group caught his hysteria, and everyone but Laura seemed to be cramming spaghetti into their mouths, diving into it with their hands, fingers, and elbows. Don, who generally held his head stiffly to one side, now threw his head back, and relaxed his throat, keeping his body soft and "open."

Brian was eating with his fingers while he meticulously tucked in the slopping overflow that, in his mind's eye, dribbled from his mouth. In between slurping and screaming, everyone was laughing so hard they almost were choking.

Laura was gradually inching her way in toward us, a small flicker of interest stirring in her green eyes.

"Could we order some escargots?" Brian asked. "They're so much more gourmet than spaghetti!"

This request set everyone off in a burst of raucous laughter.

Tears were running down Penny's cheek. "Wouldn't you know? You're such a weirdo, Brian. Escargots! What in hell is that?"

Brian, typically unruffled by such taunts, began eating his escargots. "For you, peasants, these are snails," he said.

This was too much for the group, who by now was almost completely weak with laughter. They grimaced, held their stomachs, stamped their feet, and pinched their nostrils in a unanimous signal of disapproval.

Then Laura became part of the circle, softly creeping in between Penny and me. "What do you feel like eating, Laura?" I asked. "It sounds like you could pick a dessert now, something sweet after that big meal. What would you like?"

Laura thought for a minute and then said, "Doughnuts, squishy jelly doughnuts."

"Squishy jelly doughnuts coming up!" I called with the authority of the counterclerk who knows that racks of fresh doughnuts are just out of the oven. "Here are your doughnuts, Miss," I said, presenting Laura with an imaginary box.

Laura took the imaginary box from me, opened it carefully, and passed it around to the other patients. After everyone had grabbed a doughnut, Laura carefully placed the box in the center of the circle.

"For seconds—just in case," she said. Then, to the sound of the Blood, Sweat, and Tears album, Laura began chewing and swallowing faster and faster.

"Hey, my favorite. Grape jelly. Wow!" she managed to sputter between gobbles. Laura's eyes were shining now, and her cheeks had a trace of color in them which deepened with each dive she made into the doughnut box in the center of the circle. The amazing part of Laura's mime eating was that she was using her whole body, putting her weight on one leg while extending the other upwards in the air like a ballerina. For the first time, I was able to see the spry, young girl under Laura's protective flesh.

I was surprised to see the other patients, even sophisticated Carol, still going along with the gag, jumping into the circle, grabbing the box from one another, munching, swallowing, gobbling, in an endless doughnut orgy.

But I was particularly fascinated by the movement of Laura's facial muscles. When she ate the clinic meals, she made huge quantities of food disappear vacuum cleaner-like into her mouth. The food passed through her mouth and quickly vanished, leaving Laura's facial expression unchanged. Now, although she was feverishly shoveling the imaginary doughnuts into her mouth, she actually seemed to be tasting and enjoying them. Thus, Laura, whose body temperature was generally below normal, whose hands and feet were constantly clammy and cold, and who always seemed aloof, was, at this moment, warm, alive, and responsive.

"Oops," she said, burping and giggling simultaneously, "I think I've had enough."

"Me, too," Carol said. "I can't eat another bite. How about something to wash it down with?"

"Mother's milk," Brian said, his hands upon his breast. "Mother's milk and mother's breast—the answer to the riddle."

"That and Jack Daniels on the rocks," hooted Carol.

I turned to Laura. "And for you, honey? What would you like to wash down the doughnuts?"

"A baby bottle," she said.

"OK, everybody," I said, "We've got an order from Laura for a baby bottle. I'll put on some lullabye music, while you all arrange yourselves on the floor."

I put on the Modern Jazz Quartet doing "One Never Knows," a lovely lyrical expression about a young girl.

The patients had all fallen into fetal positions, curling up naturally and spontaneously. Laura, with her thumb in her mouth, looked like a giant baby panda bear. Her position must have been identical to the one she assumed when she was ten years old, hiding under the couch in her living room, taking her baby bottle, and watching her parents dance. The thought passed through my mind that Laura would need a great amount of nurturing before she would be able to bridge her developmental gap, uncurl, and stand upright, as an independent adult.

Penny had stuck an unlit cigarette in everyone's mouth as a baby bottle substitute. I grimaced, as I realized what an on-target commentary on smoking her action was.

With her fingers protectively holding her pretend bottle, Laura's lips took on the lip-sucking motions of a small baby. Although it was Laura's idea, I couldn't help but observe the obvious satisfaction that the imaginary bottle feeding was having on the other patients. The room was quiet except for the subtle sounds of the music, and the hungry suck of baby's mouths. The taste of the wet cigarette must have been un-pleasant, and yet the dream of the bottle was strong enough to overcome any displeasure.

I waited for some kind of surfeit to set in. In a few minutes, Carol rolled over on her back, stretched, and yawned. One by one, the other patients, having had their fill, lazily straightened their legs and rolled sensuously from side to side. Laura was the last to give up the cigarette-bottle, but when she did, she too rolled over on her back, angled out her legs and draped her arms around the shoulders of Carol on one side and Kevin on the other. I got down to the floor and joined the group in a moment of relaxed daydreaming.

"Hey, this looks like what I need," said Dr. Jones, the young psychologist who worked at the clinic and who sud-denly popped his head through the door. "If you're through, we have a session coming up, and I'll want Laura and Kevin. But first I gotta stretch out. It looks too good."

The hefty little doctor let himself down gently, stretching and groaning with delight, until he had rolled alongside Don and Brian.

Dr. Jones' presence in the room was a reminder to Laura of her cardboard sign and of her responsibilities to the clinic. She rose, walked over and picked up her sign, which had been thrown on the floor by Carol, and put it around her neck.

I took Laura's hand in mine, happy to feel the unusual, pulsating warmth of her skin.

"Before you go, let's talk for a minute," I said, leading her over to the couch. Both of us settled in uncomfortably, the huge sign between us.

"Laura," I said, looking deep into her large green eyes, "do you feel full?"

Laura nodded. "I feel good," she said.

"Would you promise me something?"

"What?" she asked.

"That if you begin to have that empty feeling that you'll do some yoga breathing? Remember how it works?"

"You mean, count five, breathe in, and your stomach gets fat? Count five, breathe out, and your stomach gets thin?"

"I couldn't have said it better!" Our smiles mingled as I grabbed Laura, avoiding the sign, and rocked her. "But don't forget to let the good, clean air fill your lungs and your stomach. It may not taste as good as the real jelly doughnuts, but it may do the job as well as the pretend ones you just ate."

Laura let her head relax against me. She looked up impishly. "Do *you* do the yoga stuff?"

I nodded, "All the time."

"So then I'll just be full of hot air like you?"

"Sic transit gloria", said Dr. Jones, winking at me, as gently he led Laura and Kevin from the room.

CHAPTER III

The Cradle Rock

CAROL

With the opening beats of the acid rock that she had requested, Carol's attenuated body began its staccato movements. Her muscles moved convulsively, almost with a will of their own, as Carol became totally involved with the music. Heavy sweat covered her thin body, her nostrils were dilated, and her blue-rimmed eyes were closed, as she tossed her waist-length hair through the air. Her face was rapt, ecstatic, transported.

As I watched Carol gyrate, I reflected how, throughout history, dance has been used to relieve tensions of the body and brain. Tribal groups danced out the evil spirits with repetitive, percussive beats of their bodies. Primitive males danced to prove their virility, feeling with every flex of a muscle an affirmation of their strength. A solemn, majestic King David danced before the Lord, speaking to God for his people. The

Greeks danced their sorrows, their athletic triumphs, their ec-
stasies. In Italy, the Tarantella became a nation's convulsive
catharsis. In America, the Shakers were at one with the unities
as they vibrated into a state of grace. Turkish women belly
danced for one another, exhibiting their uncontested prowess
as females. One had only to watch Isadora Duncan's freedom
from accepted technique to be healed of one's own psychic
inhibitions. Indeed, throughout generations, unrestrained
movement, a kind of nonverbal catharsis, complete and puri-
fying, had said it all.

At the last staff meeting I had learned why Carol used
dance as her release. The daughter of wealthy, highly religious parents, she had grown up with a strong sense of guilt.
Her inordinate love for her older brother, her own deep,
unfeminine voice, her diary, discovered at a sensitive age and
its confessions laid open to mockery and suspicion—all con-
tributed to her sense of worthlessness. At fifteen, she was the
victim of a group sexual assault. Soon after, she had the first
in a series of breakdowns, was institutionalized, and for some
barbaric local reasoning, placed in solitary confinement and
forced to have her head shaved. After being released from the
institution, where the reports read that she "was much chas-
tened and subdued," she was sent away to school. In short
order she became addicted to hard drugs. For the past few
years she had been indifferently giving her body to any male
or female. Carol had begged to be whipped and beaten, for
she was filled with guilt, remorse, and self-hate. She wanted
to die as painfully as possible so that she could at least feel
something. She was twenty years old.

Carol's background seemed uncommonly significant to
me. For many of my patients with limited physical strength,

the sheer joy of healthy movement is enough to lighten their loads, at least temporarily. The intricacies of their preclinic lives, although interesting and informative, were not vital to the efficacy of a session. But with Carol, I felt I must dig into her developmental years. I had to discover why she gave her body so freely, so fully, so quickly.

Today, as our dance session progressed and I watched Carol sweat out her muscular releases, I was more than ever convinced that she wasn't dancing for pure, wholesome pleasure. Her spasms seemed designed to release some "evil" within. Though a member of the "Pepsi generation," she had the dance mania of the Middle Ages. I was no pied piper, nor was I a witch doctor who could exorcise the evil. I could only act in a limited way, as a dance therapist, and with the genuine warmth of feeling that I had acquired for this desperate girl.

Arms flailing, head down, Carol stomped furiously, even after the music had stopped. She sang in her deep voice, like an incantation, "Highs! Highs! I want 'em! I need 'em! I'm gonna get me some!" Then, with a sigh, she stopped moving and looked around her. "I can't get 'em *here,* that's for sure."

I put my hand in hers. "Carol, have you found any depths?"

Carol smiled gravely into my eyes. "Yeah, like it's a bit too deep—like over my head."

"Then let's keep it simple and uncomplicated," I suggested, "something that even a baby could understand."

For this, I put on my record of Brahm's lullaby. As the first strains of the music filled the room, Carol snickered. But within minutes she was making a cradle of her arms, her long fingers curved protectively around an imaginary baby. All of us rocked our babies with her. Penny was crooning, her skin shining with a dewy opalescence, her innocent face belying her oft-verbalized cynicism. Don held his arms out from his body so that there would be no danger of the baby touching him. Laura was amused and smiling. All of us seemed lost in the peace of an earlier day.

"Ah, to hell with this stuff," said Carol, as her deep voice rent the quiet of the nursery air. "How about cradling me?"

One aspect of working with a group is knowing when to abandon a group movement in lieu of a one-to-one encounter. At this moment I felt that there was an overriding need for Carol to have her way.

"OK, kids," I called. "Everybody pick a cradling partner."

The group split up, bewildered for a moment as I talked them into choosing partners. Laura and Brian smilingly paired up. Penny and Kevin drifted indifferently toward one another. Carol stood defiantly in front of Don until he hung his head into submission. Don, the boy who answered my question of "What do you love?" with "Math," was hardly ready for the erotic Carol. Yet, they were drawn to one another.

"OK, everybody on the floor in cradling positions!" I called, like some demented drill sergeant. I then proceeded to arrange everyone. The person doing the cradling was to sit on the floor with legs spread to accommodate the cradled person. He would then wrap his arms around his charge and rock to the lullaby music.

Carol immediately pushed Don into her lap and wrapped her long arms around him. Then her legs began a serpentine search around Don. Her pelvis was working, her face was straining, her eyes were devilishly sparkling. This was no lullaby for Carol. She was sexually maneuvering Don, who looked threatened and terrified.

"Carol, more than anything I want to see *you* being cradled," I said. "Did you forget, that's why we began this?" Seeing Don's frozen face, I added, "I think Don is the man to do it."

"Yes, yes, that would be nice," said Don, as his face relaxed somewhat with the change of plans. "I'd like to cradle Carol."

Carol was still sensuously wiggling and laughing.

"How about it, Carol? Would you like Don to be your cradler?" I asked.

Carol looked speculatively into Don's uncertain eyes. She laughed derisively. "OK, lover, let's switch."

Finally, Carol was arranged in the circle of Don's arms. There she sat, suddenly passive. A moment ago she had been all angles and wires, her hips gyrating in tightly fitted jeans, her small breasts hanging with primitive symbols. Now, quiet, she looked oddly miscast, a wan-faced rag doll, overdressed, shopworn, waiting for something to happen. Carol was not accustomed to being on the receiving end of tenderness, and the role baffled her. She had lost control of the situation.

Fortunately, Don knew about tenderness. He had abundant problems, but he *did* know about mother's love. Sweetly, he put his arms around Carol.

"You like her," I prompted Don in a whisper. "She is your friend. You don't want anything. You're not threatening her. You just want to show her how much you really like her."

Carol's body had gone quite limp. With a sigh, she sank into the circle of Don's arms. I turned up the volume on

Brahms and watched Carol rock gently in Don's embrace for a long, restful time.

When staff meetings pointed out Carol's manipulative tendencies, I went along with the suggested treatment. Carol was to continue to receive tenderness, affection, and pure friendship. In a dance-oriented situation, I was confident that I could provide the milieu for this technique. But I knew, too, that it wouldn't satisfy Carol's passionate nature, nor could it compete with the highs or the kicks that drugs and sex had previously provided for her. My plan was to give Carol her head sometimes, to let her do her Janis Joplin-like scream, but also to let her feel the physical affection and support that could come through to her if she would allow it.

"Let's form a unit, a circle unit," I said during a session. "I have a new idea for a circle game."

Everyone came swiftly into the circle. How fascinating a circle is! Comforting, sanctified, safe, we truly become a unit in joy and misery. Apes and primitive men may have formed circles for the same protective reason that we are drawn to them.

The strains of a Chopin nocturne filled the room. For a while, we simply swayed, feeling our bodies relaxing, sensing the texture and degree of intensity in our neighbors' hands.

"Squeeze hard," I suggested. "Close your eyes and see what it feels like to feel another hand tightly squeezing yours."

"Ouch!" Don cried, looking wounded. "That hurt me, Carol! That really did."

Carol snorted. "What a faggot you are!"

"Now hear this!" I called. "Loosen your grip and hold your neighbor's hand gently but firmly. Let your people know that you care, but don't break their knuckles making your point."

44

All eyes closed and smiles began to break out around the circle as patients experienced a reassuring touch.

"Now for the game. Each person will be allowed to do any physical maneuver he wants. No matter what, his partners must support him, must hold on." I looked around to see leers of mischief and expectation sprinkled on the young faces around me. "Naturally, no kicking, karate blows, biting, or rabbit punching."

This last admonition was received with wild laughter, since the battling potential of the group was fairly high.

"Me first!" Carol called. She was flanked by Don and Kevin. I knew Kevin was physically able to handle her. He was quite lucid today and interested in the game. But Don seemed far away, and I was worried that he might drop Carol's hand in a panic.

I chose a record of pagan rites, percussive and primitive. I then turned to Don and Carol.

"You're in the jungle now. You have no language," I said to Don. "But your strong arm will protect Carol." I stroked his forearm muscle admiringly.

The drums began their slow, ascending roll. The flutes wound their way seductively around the pagan melodies. Carol fairly oozed into her sensual snake dance, then she dropped to the floor. Kevin gripped hard, his face straining, his cheeks red with effort. He seemed to be enjoying the challenge. Don, on the other hand, was contorted in agony. His body had contracted. His eyes were squeezed shut. His mouth was open in terror. Yet the chain held.

"Good work, Don," I said as I passed behind him. "You can do it!"

Carol was warming to the task. Up in the air she jumped, the arms of the boys moving with her. Down she crumpled to the ground. Once again, Don and Kevin were forced to go with her, bending their knees to the fullest. Once on the floor, Carol crawled around, stretching and pawing. Then, panting, soaking wet, she stood up and with great gusto, kicked hard into the middle of the circle. One furious kick followed the other, both legs leaving the ground altogether in a moment of supreme exultation. Then, with her mouth opened wide, she threw back her head and freely screamed. Kevin and Don, still clutching Carol's hands, exchanged big grins of satisfaction.

All was quiet as Carol said, "You guys sure didn't let me down." Then she dropped her arms around both boys in a genuine gesture of affection. "Wow, what support!" she said, leaning toward Don, her head resting on his shoulder. "Never thought you had it in you, Tarzan!"

Don looked sheepishly at the floor. He blushed.

Carol walked over to me, arms outstretched. I took her into my arms and felt her body pulsate.

"Thanks," she whispered. Minutes after, Carol was gone with a brief wave of her hand.

For the dance therapist, it is strange after the emotional sound and fury of a session, to hear the sudden, abrupt silence that signals the end of the hour. Sometimes a grateful patient will stand by wistfully, wordless. There is hardly ever a traditional "Good-bye" or "Thank-you, I had a lovely time." I remember one patient who always thanked me elaborately for the lovely cha-cha lesson, which was, I suppose, his cover for the screaming, crawling session he generally had. Another woman treated me as the Arthur Murray instructor at what she firmly believed to be a Catskill resort. She never missed kissing me au revoir quite theatrically while she gasped out how divine the dance lesson had been.

But for the most part, a therapist doesn't expect formalities, nor does she want the patient to evaluate the session. She does hope desperately that the patient has internalized something of his experience. For in any session, emotions are released that are hard to evaluate or chart. How could one, for example, measure the efficacy of Carol's release, or the healthiness of her spontaneous hug? Hopefully, when Carol walked back to her cottage today, she carried something of a special nature that only dance therapy could provide for her.

CHAPTER IV

The Wall of Life

BRIAN

I use only two trusty, "structured" techniques in my dance therapy sessions: the circle formation and a dancer's warm-up exercises. I direct the warm-up exercises, some of which are foolproof tension-dispellers. I tell the patients to rotate their heads, shrug their shoulders, and stretch their arms first to the ceiling and then to the walls. I try to get them to bend their knees and let their torsos sag forward. I coax them to shake their fingers limp, roll their eyes, yawn, breathe deeply, and feel the space around them. Some of the patients with memories of high school gym classes or life at boot camp seem to enjoy the structure of disciplined exercise. Others despise the movements and are uncooperative, and it is with them that I become a dance therapist immediately, my eye alert for movements or lack of movements to clue me in on a particular problem. Beginning dance therapists often find this need to watch exhausting, yet it is an essential part of dance therapy.

I like my patients to go barefoot so that they can actually feel the ground beneath them. Many of my men and women patients tread the ground so lightly, so tentatively, that you sense their fear and repugnance for touching a base as primitive as Mother Earth. My way of handling this is very direct:

"Toss your shoes over there," I say, pointing to an unused area of the room, "and pull your socks off!"

"Must I?" asks Don, as he watches the group remove their shoes. "It's so rotten filthy in here."

"C'mon, just try it, Don," I say.

Don looks intently down at his work boots. "Well, do you mind if I clean the floor first? This place is a pig pen!"

"OK, give it a fast brush and come back to us. We need you."

Don tucks his shirt in meticulously, straightens his belt buckle, rubs the palms of his hands together, stoops for another swipe at his boots, and then goes off purposefully to the broom closet.

Meanwhile, the group warms up, stretching, yawning, becoming aware of forgotten parts of their bodies. Carol stretches and then shrugs her shoulders, once, twice, three times, her face impassive.

"How's that feel to you, Carol?" I ask, shrugging along with her.

Carol lifts her shoulders almost to her ears. "Like I don't care. Like I just don't care," she says.

"I don't care," Laura repeats softly, as we all shrug away to the sound of the Roaring Twenties' jazz beat, a musical request of Brian's. "I don't care," Laura drones on, "so bug off, you bastards!"

This surprise ending tickles Penny, who adores profanity. "Good Christ, that's great!" she howls. "Bug off, you bastards!" Penny widens her shrug into an aggressive arm movement and jabs an elbow into Don, who is just returning to the group, having cleaned his spot in the room.

Don grunts in pain, purses his lips in disapproval, and wrinkles his nose as if he had smelled a foul odor.

"Why do you let her do that to you, Don?" I ask. "Why don't you tell Penny to bug off?"

Don's eyes suddenly fill with tears.

"Well, tell her with your body, then," I suggest.

Very gently, gingerly, Don prods Penny with his elbow.

Penny jumps back in exaggerated terror. "Ooooh, you're real scary, Don baby. You're a regular tiger!"

Don blushes and grins. He takes a small, shy step sidewise in Penny's direction, and suddenly, although the session is only a few minutes old, body interplay has begun. As Don impulsively pulls off his shoes, I look around sharply to see what the others are saying through movement. Laura's fingers seem to be groping for something; I bring her Kevin's hands, followed by his somewhat reluctant body. I can feel only a modicum of resistance, so I know it is a safe gesture for him to make, and for me to encourage. I am vindicated for Kevin sighs as his hands touch Laura's. She grins. Penny's head seems to be inclining toward some safe harbor. I manage to wheedle Don into lending a shoulder, which is not difficult, since he has inched up to Penny gradually after their initial body contact. I am also there to exchange a full, free smile with Carol, whose glacially set features of a few minutes ago have just melted.

Using Don's shoulder as a "barre," Penny has just succeeded in balancing herself on one leg, while thrusting the other straight behind her like a ballet dancer. Her departure from her habitual posture (in Penny's case, her legs are usually held tensely and tightly together) seems to generate a release of tension, followed by an emotionally charged reaction. Thus, I am prepared for Penny's sudden fit of sobbing. My arms go around her trembling body for immediate, unmistakable support. Don, looking somewhat dazed, gently pats Penny on the back.

So far, so good. There is movement. There is progress. There are discoveries. However, no dance therapist can afford to think that her skills will affect all members of the group simultaneously. There is at least one patient who defies you, who distrusts you, who fights you.

For me, it is Brian who is the hardest to reach. Tall, dark, electrifyingly intense, he dances to his own music, beats his own body masochistically like a drum. His dances have no beginning, no middle, no end. They are short, angry bursts of attack. He refuses to be questioned, interpreted, or structured. When we form a circle, he will run, skip, and leap around its periphery. Sometimes I will join him in his animated leaping, fascinated as I watch his feet hit his buttocks like some woodland animal. For a moment, as our strides match and our rhythms mesh, he looks down at me with recognition and joy. But the moment passes, and he is off again to his private world.

Brian is usually the first to arrive in the recreation room, a sign of enthusiasm that he would no doubt deny. He is usually dressed in a threadbare plaid shirt, beltless khaki pants, and a thick, vintage college sweater, yellowed, raveled, and shrunken. He seems to endure calmly the weight of his clothing on his thin, fiery frame. But in spite of the tattered, unprotected image he projects, he is a totally armored man.

Before his twelve years in various mental institutions, Brian was the typical Ivy League hero. He had been a prep school leader and a top college athlete. While being trained as a jet pilot, however, Brian had his first breakdown. The perfect American boy sank into apathy, his former glories forgotten. Friends and family stood by in shock, powerless to help. Nor could the many institutions in which Brian was subsequently placed find the reason for his apathy.

Brian was a mystifying and challenging wisp of a man when his parents brought him to our clinic ten years ago. Whatever strength he could marshal seemed to be channeled into his desire to die. Initially, a marathon effort was made by the medical director and therapists merely to keep Brian alive. He was spoon fed and bottle fed around the clock. Then the clinic staff tried to fan some small flame of hope in Brian's broken body by trying to get him to share his misery. It was hard going. Complete despair engulfed him. He could not talk, walk, or even move an eyelash. He could barely eat or defecate. But slowly, with infinite care and love and endless patience on the part of the staff, Brian decided to live.

Six years later, I joined the clinic and found thirty-five-year-old Brian a strange, withdrawn man with a young, boyish face, a contracted body posture, and a defenseless smile that went right to my heart. He functioned well, although somewhat automatically. Yet when Brian danced, he was as free as a wild bird.

In the session today, Brian seemed to be watching us as we threw our heads back, exposing our throats. Patients who

53

habitually duck their heads to protect an exposure of this vulnerable area find this movement difficult. Narrowing his eyes like an artist surveying his work, Brian says, "I see some proud horses."

"Will you join the herd?" I ask.

Brian steps back a pace or two. He tucks his head toward his chest, crumples his abdomen, and turns his bent knees in toward one another. "How's this for pride?" he smirks.

"Hey, Brian" Carol says, peering up into Brian's hidden face, "we put this crummy music on for you. Why'n hell don't you move?"

Brian responds to Carol's challenge by straightening up and kicking his legs high and fast in an animated Charleston.

I dance over to him and kick along with him. Suddenly, he wheels around and aims a kick at me, but checks it before it lands.

"Was that for me, Brian?" I ask.

Brian's eyes flash with fury. He's breathing hard. "I rarely kick when I'm angry," he says. "I prefer at that time to make a fraudulent gesture like this!" He angrily snaps his fingers hard under my nose, his nail scraping my skin. As I flinch, Brian's eyes soften and he put his hand on my shoulder.

"I'm sorry, Helene," he says, reaching for an unaccustomed intimacy with me. "I'm angry at the wall of life behind you."

"The wall of life?" I said.

I turned around to see the pale blue, accordian-pleated vinyl curtain that we use as a room divider. Fastened to two posts and nine feet wide, the curtain runs along a track across the ceiling and locks shut with a metal device at one end.

Brian points to the curtain, saying in a prophetic manner:

"Behind that wall there is love, warmth, and companionship." "Here," his arms defined our side of the room, "are the mad wanderings of my mind."

The jazz record had finished playing. Quickly, I put on a Debussy record—"Prelude to the Afternoon of a Faun." At the first strains of the music, Brian places his back to "the wall." Suddenly, Brian contracts his body and inclines his head toward his chest as he falls to the floor in a fetal position. The other patients are swaying gently to the music, arms intertwined, watching very quietly as Brian responds with his body to the alternatives: life, behind the curtain; death, on our side of the room.

For a moment, Brian remains locked in his fetal position. Then, gradually, slowly, he begins rocking and crawling, pushing and tearing at the space around him. He presses forward, and then falls backward. He rolls over, sighs, and then groans. Brian seems lost in his perilous quest. Then, with enormous effort, he pulls himself up to a kneeling position. Still on his knees, he drags himself across the floor where he focuses intently on the curtain. He touches the folds with inquisitive fingers, and then, suddenly as if it were too hot to handle, his hand falls away, as Brian turns sharply from the curtain, falling back once again into a fetal position.

"No! No! Brian," Penny screams, pulling at his contracted body. "No! You didn't try hard enough to get through the wall." Penny, who had once tried to end her life with a knife, did not want Brian to choose death over life. Yet while Brian preferred to live in his subconscious, Penny barely acknowledged hers. Like a boxer, Penny began flailing away at Brian.

"Let me show you how to beat the crap out of that life wall!" Penny shrieks.

There was a kaleidoscopic display of colors as Penny's long, dark, curly gypsy hair mixed with her long red skirt and her purple shirt. She began beating at the curtain with her fists.

"You rotten, stinking wall, I'll get through! I'll make it!" And with that, she pummeled the wall with all of her one hundred pounds. Suddenly, the curtain buckled under her fierce assault, as folds of it collapsed around Penny's head and shoulders. Penny began laughing and crying under the weight of it.

"Look at me, the crazy madonna!" she said, squinting up at me, "but goddamn, I got a good look at life, didn't I?"

I got down on my knees then and put my arms around Penny, curtain and all. "You fought your way through the wall, didn't you?"

Penny laughed. "That's no friggin' trick. I've been doing that all my life. I guess I got Mom's crummy temper."

"Well, you certainly made a spectacle of yourself!" Don said, approaching Penny with a shy, sidewise movement that belied his sharp tongue.

Penny looked up angrily, defensively. "OK, smart ass, you got any better ideas?"

Don began to chew his fingernails as he pondered her question. "Yeah, I think I do," he finally mutters.

"All right," I said, "we have another contender for the wall of life. Let's straighten the curtain and give Don a little room."

I help Penny off the floor and onto the couch where she collapses, spent and wet with perspiration, beside Brian. She puts her head on Brian's shoulder. The other patients stand by, eyeing Don skeptically as he stalks up to the curtain.

Don, slight, blond, so neat that he gives the impression of being stapled together, has a robotlike quality. Now, he further tucks in the shirt that never was untucked, brushes the dust off his spotlessly clean pants, and rubs his pale hands together. Then, meticulously, he begins rehanging the curtain, taking particular care that each fold is even with the next.

"Jesus, if I had to worry about such perfection, I'd kill myself . . . again," Penny says, as a look of comprehension flooded her face. "What was the use anyway? I could never do anything as good as my sister! Except some things. . . ." She snuggles into Brian with a look of pure deviltry shining in her eyes.

Debussy plays on, as Don slowly paces the length of the curtain. With exquisite care, his fingers run up and down each fold. Standing on his toes, he strains to examine the top of the wall. He does a knee bend to his haunches as he peers beneath the curtain. With a face full of mischief, he faces us, his audience. Suddenly, unable to contain his excitement, he jumps in the air and kicks his heels together, like a Russian folk dancer. Then, in unbearable delight, he stomps out a little ecstatic jig. A true showman, Don changes pace and soberly bows to us. With his hands well-hidden behind him, he deftly presses the lock opening. As the curtain parts, Don turns sharply, and with sure, giant strides marches through to the other side.

In response to the enthusiastic applause he receives from Kevin, Laura, and me, Don expansively holds out his nail-bitten fingers.

"Golden hands," he says, "golden hands is what my father said God gave him. He could do anything with them. He said I was like my mother's side. All thumbs!" Don laughs.

"Whose side do you think you're on now, Don?" I ask.

"Nobody's. I want to be on my own side," Don says, looking down at his hands, "but . . . I like my hands golden."

"Wow, you were like something on the TV," Laura gushes. "You should be in the movies, Don."

Penny hoots. "Yeah, you could play some small-town, rip-off guy. Why can't you bust through that wall like a man . . . with a roar?" Penny makes a little contemptuous sound with her lips.

Brian is stimulated. "Yes, of course, a roar. Like a tethered lion by the light of the moon."

Don laughs. "A fat chance I'd have getting through that wall with a roar!"

Penny challenges him again. "I like my men with some guts. You're really such a faggot."

Don's color heightens. "If you weren't a girl, I'd punch you right in the nose."

At this, Penny jumps off the couch, ready for a fight. "Try me, just try, right there!" she teases, pointing to her chin.

Brian comes between them. He likes Don and is attracted to him. He puts his arms around him. "Would you like to hear me roar, Don?"

Don grins. "Yeah."

Brian then gets down on all fours, sticks his tongue out, and roars a free, deep, male lion's roar.

Had Brian been a therapist, he couldn't have planned a better mood change. Don is frankly admiring, and in minutes the group is roaring. Don's choked, little throat sound now mingles with Kevin's chimpanzee hoot-pant. Penny grabs the bongos, and suddenly a real jungle beat is established.

Our session ended in an African war dance and a spontaneous release of the tension that Brian's "wall of life" built up for all of us.

When I described this dance therapy session to the therapists at the weekly staff meeting, they were amazed at Brian's performance. The therapists had observed Brian in many different activities, playing in ball games, talking rationally on the telephone, even attempting to fall in love with a female patient. Yet in dance therapy Brian's behavior had been totally bizarre. Did dance therapy encourage him to turn from reality?

Though our discussion about Brian's performance was a curious mixture of Jungian, Freudian, Adlerian, Behaviorist, and Gestalt thought, we all agreed that Brian seemed to love dancing. Since it was obviously an excellent release for him, it was decided that dance therapy should continue to be part of Brian's program.

It was also decided at the meeting that I would henceforth have a permanent assistant dance therapist, Dr. Jones. This young clinical psychologist was not a stranger to me. On the contrary, he had attended a few dance therapy sessions with enthusiasm. I was elated to have him assigned this way, for I knew that our dance therapy sessions would benefit by his on-the-spot psychological insights. I was also grateful to the clinic for providing me with this kind of support. If a dance therapist is forced to go through her paces with a patient as if there were no yesterday or no tomorrow, with no briefing before and no follow-up later, she might well question her efforts. For pure release, why not basketball or volleyball? The fact that my colleagues recognized that my working in a vacuum would be an injustice to my patients and to me further deepened my love for the clinic.

"I need the exercise," Dr. Jones said, patting his rounded abdomen. "Think I can lose some of this in your dance therapy sessions?"

"I'll promise you a lost pound for every psychological insight gained," I said.

I looked forward to having this young man work with me, and hoped that together we might discover some new directions for dance therapy.

CHAPTER V

The Day They Clobbered The Dance Therapist

KEVIN

One day, I appeared for a dance therapy session and found the patients tense and surly.

"Here comes the goddamn she-bitch," Don said, as I walked into the room.

"You really think I'm a bitch, Don?" I asked.

"Yeah," Don said, hitching up his pants, his pale skin coloring with anger, "yeah, you really stink. Christ, you were a 'no show' last week."

"Well, I was sick last week—but I'm here now."

Don looked straight at me with a sneer on his face. Then he blinked his eyes nervously and raised his arm as if to strike me. Knowing how indecisive Don is, I was fairly certain that he would not physically attack me. But nonetheless, I was wary as I backed away.

Although a dance therapist cannot work in constant fear of an assault, she must be prepared for a sudden blow, a hard jab, or some other unexpected physical expression of a patient's hostility. Sometimes the therapist's faulty or insensitive technique may precipitate a patient's attack. But more often, an assault can be the result of a successful transference on the part of the patient, so that in many instances, the dance therapist becomes the patient's "mother." Sometimes even a healthy child who wants more attention from his mother will make his demands in a negative way. He may use unacceptable language, or even poke an elbow into mommy's eyes as she bends down for a kiss. It is not surprising, therefore, to find a mental patient asking for love in similar devious ways.

As I backed away from Don's threatening arm, I remembered an assault incident that occurred early in my career when I was neither watchful nor knowledgeable. I was conducting my class in a locked ward of a state hospital. My twenty top-security patients were remarkably submissive, especially when one considered their turbulent histories, but daily tranquilizers had most of them yawning and spiritless. Dance therapy for this listless bunch was an exercise in sleep-walking to music.

As a novice, I was dedicated to the theory that an instantaneous response from my patients would insure my success with them. Since gentle music seemed to bring on an epidemic of yawning, I had stocked the record player with some wild, African tribal music. I was thrilled to see some impulsive stomping movement by several members of the group. However, in a corner, by herself, stood a tremendous woman, at least six feet tall, who was paying little attention to the group, the music, or me. I had turned my attention to the stomping patients, when suddenly I heard the sound of scuffling behind me. One of the patients who had been dancing near the corner was screaming and holding her reddened cheek. Apparently, the tall, seemingly diffident woman had smacked her in the face for no apparent reason and was now blithely jiggling around to the music, though her fists were still clenched. I comforted the victim, who was more surprised than hurt, as I watched her assailant dance by, her fists swinging ominously.

The record then changed to Miriam Makeba's quieter South African songs. "There's a flea in my hair," sang Miss Makeba, and everyone seemed settled and amused. As I danced around the circle, facing each patient for some individual hand contact, I suddenly felt someone's presence behind me, followed by a light pressure on my head. For one brief moment, hypnotized by the music, I wondered whether in fact someone *was* putting a flea in my hair. Then, remembering where I was, I whirled around aggressively to confront the six-foot face-smacker, who did indeed have her hand on my head. However, it was the other hand I should have worried about. Startled by my sudden move, she aimed a barrelhouse wallop at my nose. I saw it coming and grabbed on to her swinging fist with both my hands. In a moment, she had swung me around ninety-degrees, so that I was now nose to nose with her murderous face. Instead of calling for an attendant or attempting to free myself, I foolishly continued to be the dedicated young therapist.

"Let's dance it out," I gasped as I spun through the air. In point of fact, I was already dancing, my buckling knees unwittingly doing a South African native dance, though somewhat above the floor, as I continued to cling like a leech to the woman's fist.

The ludicrous situation apparently struck my giant assailant as wildly hilarious. With great whoops of laughter, she began to dance, letting me down abruptly to the floor, and propelling me in what was probably an original in the annals of South African tribal rites.

The rest of the patients stood by awestruck, watching the floor show. When the record ended, the performers—my six-foot dancing partner and I—bowed to unrestrained applause. My tall partner was ready for another number, but in deference to my trembling knees, I announced that the session was now officially over. My patients returned to their quarters chattering enthusiastically about the dance therapy session, while I, in turn, leaned weakly against the wall, soaking wet and exhausted. I knew then that I had learned forever to be alert to the meaning of a dangerously clenched fist, and that a patient's light touch on my head might or might not be pure affection. But more to the point, I had learned not to turn my back on any member of a group for more than a few seconds.

That incident took place several years ago. Today, I take my cues more rapidly. After I had cautiously ducked away from Don, I walked toward the record player and put on a restful Viennese waltz. My patients gathered for the opening circle, Kevin on my left, frowning and unyielding, but holding my hand firmly. On my right was soft, round Laura, giving me a mechanical, bland smile, while she took my hand. She then proceeded to bend my fingers back painfully, all the while smiling at me. At this stage of my development as a dance therapist, I knew enough to distrust the smile and react to the fierce finger-pressure message, but my knowledge did not ease the pain in my hand.

I turned my face toward Laura's. "Let's dance this waltz together, just you and me," I said, breathing easier as Laura's grip on my fingers relaxed.

I looked around the circle to see who was lucid and approachable. "Carol, would you start Kevin and Brian and the others in some loosening-up exercise?"

Carol's eyes looked somewhat glazed, but the position of leadership was one she enjoyed, however briefly. While she was weighing the lure of controlling the group against the counter-lure of her apathy, Kevin dropped my hand and turned from the circle. Not willing to let him go yet, I quickly grabbed his hand and attached it to Brian's. "Stay here with Kevin and Carol," I said in Brian's ear. "I'll be back in a jiffy."

Carol had made her decision. She was standing in the center of the circle, issuing orders.

"OK, you guys, I want you to relax . . . and fast!" Carol led the way by slowly rotating her head on her long, slim neck, as her silky dark hair flipped forward and covered her face.

Now I could safely turn my full attention to Laura. She stood with her feet slightly apart, her short block of a body defying me to move her.

I leaned close to her. "OK, Laura, lead me anywhere you want. Make me do anything you like. You will be the leader, and I will follow you anywhere." I looked into her large green eyes and gently pinched her small freckled nose. "I am in your power," I said, in my best "Count Dracula" voice.

Laura smirked at my performance. She put her hands on my shoulder. "Close your eyes, Mrs. Lefco. Go ahead. I won't hurt you."

At this moment of truth, I *half*-closed my eyes. I trust some of my patients—Laura more than most—but not all of them.

Laura then moved me backwards, aggressively, as her feet slid forward in waltz time. She led me in a strong, yet unviolent way, with a sustained movement in a direction clearly defined by her. Laura's pudgy fingers dug into my skin as we danced, until suddenly, she had backed me into a corner. I then pretended to collapse, my head down, my shoulders dispirited.

"Is this where you want me, Laura? In the dunce corner?" I asked.

Laura nodded. "Yeah, 'cause you're a dunce." She watched me closely through narrowed eyes as I stayed plastered to the corner, my body meek and submissive.

"You didn't come last week, did you?" she asked.

"No, Laura, I had a sore throat, and I didn't want to give it to you."

"Were your children home with you?"

"No," I answered carefully, suspecting sibling rivalry. "They were all at school." I raised my head and looked into Laura's suspicious eyes. "Did you miss me?"

Laura nodded gravely.

"I really wanted to come, Laura, but the doctor didn't think it was a good idea."

Laura breathed heavily as she assessed my sincerity. Satisfied, she nodded, and put out her hand.

"OK, you can come out of the corner now." This time her handclasp was gentle and warm. Hand in hand we returned to the circle.

Carol was still tossing her hair around with obvious enjoyment, but no one else seemed to be moving. Apparently after her opening salvo, Carol's interest in leading the group had gone steadily downhill, and now her self-absorption had set her charges totally adrift. The group was standing around lifelessly and with the remoteness of children who feel no one cares.

Penny suddenly burst into the room, ten minutes late. She walked quickly and stiffly past all of us, her head down, her chest concave. I put my hand out to her.

"Take your friggin' hand offa me," she said, as she stormed over to the couch and threw herself upon it. "I feel lousy."

In a second, her soft, small, feline face became a blank mask of indifference.

Noting the unusually withdrawn mood of the group, my usual opening swings and stretches seemed too tame, too unchallenging. I put on Elizabeth Waldo's "Rites of the Pagan," a wildly creative musical exploration into ancient Indo-American civilization. Perhaps this primitive theme, the battle of a serpent with an eagle, and the accompanying sound of drums, recorders, double flutes, and whistles might receive a spontaneous response from the group. Glancing around the room eagerly for a reaction to the music, I found that, unfortunately, I was the only one inspired to move.

I resolved to go another round. There are days like this!

"OK," I said to the group, "I'm going to shout out a word and see how fast you can react to it with your body."

"Oh, God, not that crap, again," Penny said, flouncing off the couch. "I'm going to beat the drums while you play

your games, though I'm not so friggin' fond of that either!"
she muttered.

Her small, vividly painted mouth set grimly, Penny ran
off to get the big drum which she used as counterpoint to the
music of the record. I listened intently to the music, and at the
same time combed the room with my eyes for any movement
that I could expand upon and translate into a word that would
ignite my patients' desire to move.

"Anybody got an idea for a word?" I asked, stalling for
time. "Could it be 'snake' . . . 'slippery' . . .," and then added,
influenced by the serpentine theme of the music, " 'Twisting,'
'evil,' 'predatory' . . .?"

Don lunged forward toward me. "What the hell is this
supposed to be? A goddamn spelling bee?"

I lunged back at him, and the word I was seeking flew
into my head—"revenge." The patients were furious because
I disappointed them last week by being absent, and now they
were paying me back for my neglect. They were deliberately
avoiding my musical cues. Today, they wanted things done
their way.

"The magic word is 'revenge,' " I shouted.

The word hung in the air for seconds. I watched, fascinated, as it drifted like a cloud around the faces of the patients. Laura smiled like a cat licking her chops. Penny's eyes
burned with an impish delight. Carol stroked her long hair as
if limbering her fingers for action.

"Yah! Yah!" Brian ran with an imaginary sword pointed
straight to my throat. Don charged in after Brian, screaming,
"Revenge! Revenge is sweet!" Brian and Don were like two
warriors now, two musketeers, although Brian's fighting position was somewhat unorthodox. His half-cocked arm was
thrust forward, while his other arm reached backward, his

fingers outstretched. The main thrust of Brian's ferocity was in his scowling face, but his knees were bent, and he had an unaccustomed look of agility about him. Both men were grunting with effort, their mouths open and free. All around the room patients were acting out personal motifs of revenge. Laura and Carol were grappling, their fingers around each other's necks, their faces flushed with the excitement of battle. Penny was shrieking a war cry in between fevered drum beats.

"Kill 'em! Get 'em! Get your red-hot revenge while it lasts! Squeeze 'em! Whack 'em! Slice 'em! Yahoo—it's a goddamn riot!"

Accompanying this dramatic outburst was the considerably milder sound of tribal rites still coming from the record player.

Unable to contain herself any longer, Penny threw down the drum and came hunting for me. With great gusto she jabbed me with her hip and shoulder. I jabbed back with my shoulder, not as strongly, but with conviction. We played the body-bumping game of my childhood, hopping on one foot, crashing into one another with force.

In the middle of this brouhaha, a quiet little vignette was taking place. Dr. Jones, my assistant, was trying to goad Kevin into moving, or, at the very least, into reacting.

"C'mon, Kevin, don't I look like your brother, Lenny? He was the favorite, wasn't he? Everybody liked Lenny, didn't they, Kevin? C'mon, get mad, Kevin! The girls really went for Lenny, didn't they, Kevin? Kevin, whaddya gonna do about Lenny?"

Kevin usually appeared physically paralyzed, but his mumbling was nonstop. Very rarely did he speak in a direct way, though his coded mumbling was loaded with meaning once one learned to discount two out of three of his

69

sentences. His feet were normally glued to the ground, his knees tense and stiff. Yet as I watched, Kevin's shoulders suddenly shot up and his eyes began to dart about the room. One side of his face was twitching.

Brian was watching with interest as Dr. Jones tried to get the reluctant Kevin to react to his suggestions. For many years, Brian had been in Kevin's immobilized condition. To get Brian moving in those dark days, a battery of psychiatric techniques had been unleashed on him. For Brian, this scene between Dr. Jones and Kevin must have touched a nerve, or perhaps started him projecting. Then, suddenly, with fists clenched, teeth gritted, and arms cocked in fighting position, Brian approached Kevin.

"OK, you lazy bastard. Move. Get on with it. What do you think this is? A goddamn mental institution? Are you God or something? Get on with it, Kevin boy!" and then, as an afterthought, "And tell your voices to bug off!"

Brian's tirade had been made in a low, animal snarl, gutteral and coarse, a far cry from his usual, somewhat high-pitched, effeminate voice. His right arm drew back in preparation for a punch. At this point, however, Brian checked himself, pulled half-way back, and struck Kevin with a weak, ineffectual blow.

All of Brian's movements reduced him to a treadmill of motion. When he ran, one leg shot forward, the other pushed backward. When his head and torso were forward, his lower half seemed to be pulling in the other direction. When he moved one arm in an Australian crawl stroke, the other arm held him stationary with a backstroke. When he kicked his legs forward, his toes turned up, bent almost backward.

70

The Day They Clobbered the Dance Therapist

Observing Brian's bizarre movements, I am reminded of the Air Force's comparison of their novice pilots to the kiwi bird. The Air Force pilots say that the kiwi bird flies backward because he is not interested in where he is going, but rather, in where he has been. He flies backward in ever decreasing spirals, until he flies up his own rectum and disappears.

Kevin, ignoring the force of Brian's outburst, merely replied with another spate of mumbling. Then his vibrating body jerked him loose from his spot on the floor, and he began to stagger toward the door. Dr. Jones, however, was ready to "talk" him back.

"Oh, so you are just going to walk away from Brian's stuff, are you? You're just going to let him punch you anytime he pleases, is that it? Isn't that what your brother has been doing to you all these years, giving you a good jerking around any time he's in the mood?"

Kevin looked frightened. Raised as a Southern gentleman, he generally tried to be mannerly and soft-spoken. But now, he was completely cowed by Dr. Jones and Brian. His eyes teared. His mouth trembled. His lips continued to form incoherent words, as his arms flapped up and down against his sides in impotent despair. Kevin's tall, thin frame, elongated further by his heavy, high-heeled cowboy boots, seemed to be tautly pulled inward at the middle as he slinked away from Brian. His eyes sought me out, as he desperately looked around for help.

"Who are *you?*" he asked. "The football coach? The dancing teacher?" Then his eyes lit on my sweater, and he looked away nervously. "You got your bumps on. Are you my mother? Is it safe? Can I talk?"

Imploringly, Kevin faced Brian. "Are you my girl friend? Am I the girl? Are you the boy? Who am I?"

Brian seemed moved by this. Immediately, he dropped his aggressive stance and put his arms around Kevin. Face to face, he wordlessly embraced Kevin—and Kevin, with a deep sigh, hugged back.

As I watched the scene taking place, it was hard to believe that Kevin's clinging, weaving, uncertain figure had the violence within it to have almost killed a man with a golf club.

Suddenly, from the record player, a blast of full volume rock sound shook the room. Carol was dancing around gleefully, moving her pelvis like a belly dancer. "I thought we could use a little action, man. This place is getting awful heavy." Carol inclined her head in the direction of Dr. Jones and Kevin. "Who needs that stuff? It really freaks me out. What we need are the Stones, man."

The Rolling Stones, a rock group alive with a frank sexuality that it projects at a consistent fevered pitch, completely destroyed the more creative mood that the tribal rites music had engendered. Like mechanical wind-up dolls programmed to respond to the sound of the peer-group beat, the group came shaking and jerking into the center of the room, close to one another, but maintaining a sense of separateness. Brian had left Kevin's side and was now leaping through the air. Even hefty Dr. Jones had thrown himself in with the group and was moving his hips awkwardly but happily. Suddenly Kevin, too, jumped up into the air like a young Masai warrior, high, stiff, in one piece, with enormous elevation. Fascinated by Kevin's African jumps, I got closer and jumped along with him. One jump, two jumps, and we were together in the air.

And then, in one, swift, mystifying moment, I was swooped up, sent spiraling through space, and propelled downward until I hit the cement floor.

My initial awareness as I lay there on the floor was not so much of pain, but rather of complete surprise. Having never played football, basketball, or any contact sport that would regularly have exposed me to a sudden fall, I was amazed by the abrupt sound and feeling of bone and flesh on cement. As I mused on this phenomenon, the patients gathered around me, stunned. Kevin was the closest down on his knees, peering into my face.

"I didn't mean it, Mrs. Lefco, I'm sorry," he cried. "I thought you were big, strong, like a football coach. C'mon, hit me! Hit me! It's your turn. Knock me down. It's OK. You can knock me down." Tears spilled down over his face. "I'm sorry."

Much as my head hurt, I was tremendously impressed by the sincerity, coherency, and lack of mumbling in Kevin's speech. I used one hand to feel the bump on my head, and put my other hand on Kevin's arm.

"I'm OK, Kevin, I'm really OK."

Inexplicably, Don was now sobbing. "He didn't do it. I did it. I didn't want to, but it just came over me. Mama's dead. Look at her. Dead." Don's hands covered his face and he sobbed.

I could no longer rub my head. There were more important things to do with my hands. My arms went around Don as he bent over me, sobbing.

"Everbody wants to take a poke at mama, Don. Don't worry about it. Except that *you* didn't do it this time," I said.

Brian also peered down at me, his face perplexed. "This is a pickle. I'd really like to know. Who did it? Did I?" And then Brian turned questioningly to Dr. Jones, who was kneeling beside me with the rest of the group. "Did you do it?"

This struck me funny, and as I laughed, the fright left my body. When I thought of all the questioning going on as to who had perpetrated the foul deed, I began to feel like the hero Robin, in "Who Killed Cock Robin?," and this made me laugh even harder. One look at Dr. Jones' serious face made me suspect that he thought I was becoming hysterical. Gently, he began to help me to my feet. "Think you can make it, Helene?"

I rubbed my head, flexed my back, wiggled my body a bit, and then decided that my years of practicing dance falls had not been in vain. Instinctively, I had protected myself by landing on all of the soft spots, except for my head. In my bleary state, I recognized that my injury was no more than a slight concussion.

"Get the derrick and pull me up, Jones," I said as he propped me up to a standing position.

Kevin was now completely hysterical, babbling, crying in a high-pitched, childish voice. Dr. Jones quickly led him out of the room, back to his quarters. Over his shoulder, Kevin's tear-stained face looked back at me.

"Can I ever come back to dancing class?" he called out.

"I hope so, Kevin," I said. And then, pointing to my head, "That is, if I can count on *this* not happening again!"

"It wasn't supposed to happen *this time,* Mrs. Lefco!" Kevin said.

I grinned with pure joy. Kevin had answered with humor, clarity, directness. I shook my throbbing head. It was too bad I couldn't employ this technique more often to elicit a clear response from Kevin.

Don was at my side. "So Kevin did it, did he? I hate him. What a disgusting beast!"

Carol was patting my shoulder. "What a bunch of finks in this place. I really hate everyone's guts!"

Laura walked up to me shyly. "You OK? Does your head hurt bad?" she asked anxiously.

I put my arms around Laura's thick waist. "I'm fine."

Laura put her arm through mine. "It was like you were my sister. Like sometimes, when I was young, I really wanted to floor her. But it really scared me when I saw you lying there."

Brian had been standing thoughtfully by listening to Laura. Now he spoke in a quiet, matter-of-fact voice.

"I guess it's all over now . . .all the dancing. The music will stop, eh?"

I then took my first steps since my fall and was relieved to know that all my parts were still functioning. "Brian, I'm going to put a record on now, and I hope to put on ten thousand more for dance therapy sessions." Smiling at him, I added, "I've got a tough noggin."

Brian sighed and put his arms around me, but at the same time, he managed to wind his body away from me. Perhaps our respective roles in the drama that had just unfolded had been too much for him. As I watched, he left me, mind, spirit, and body. But once again, characteristically, Brian could not consolidate all of himself. Although his legs and torso were moving away from me, his head was still turned in my direction.

"What did you say your name was?" he asked.

I put on John Williams' record of "Two Guitar Concertos," and the sound of pastoral musical poetry filled the room. Soothed and quieted, we all settled down on the carpeted area of the room. My head dropped contemplatively on my chest, but my mind anxiously returned to the question of why Kevin had chosen the moment when I was mirroring his high jumps to forcibly push me away.

Dr. Jones, back in the recreation room after escorting Kevin to his quarters, joined our group. He sprawled comfortably on the red carpet with us to discuss the incident.

"I think Kevin was confused, Helene," he said. "Brian had just caressed him, and he felt himself warmly responding. Right on the heels of this encounter, you arrive, literally jumping up at him with passion. He likes you. You are many women to him. His sister, his mother, his girl friend. Think of it. What a bind for a confused boy like Kevin to have responded to Brian's homosexual advance and to be almost immediately tempted by a heterosexual possibility." Dr. Jones shook his head. "I think it was simply too much for him to handle. Kevin had to push something away," he said frowning, "and unfortunately, it was you. I might have precipitated it," Dr. Jones continued, "by trying to release some of his anger." He laughed, gently rubbing my head, "I hadn't figured that he'd work it out on *you*."

Thinking about what Dr. Jones had said, I settled back in a crossed-leg yoga position, and took some deep breaths. Oh well, it wasn't all bad. I looked around at the patients. Their faces were peaceful. Don and Laura had dealt with "Mom" and "Sis" and knocked both of them down summarily. Carol and Penny had shown tenderness and concern. Even Brian had made it through his miasma of confusion, if only for a few minutes. Kevin had organized and spoken his thoughts precisely. On balance, I think I was glad the incident had happened. As if reading my mind, Carol pointed toward my head.

"Your dance therapy lumps are showing, Mrs. Lefco," Carol said. "I guess even *you* don't know all the answers."

"You can say that again!" I laughed, taking Carol's hand. She in turn brought Brian into our sitting circle, while he stretched out an arm to Don, Laura, and Penny. All of us were together, our arms around one another, our bare toes touching, one head inclined toward the other. As the session closed, we hummed and swayed to the sound of guitars.

CHAPTER VI

Dance Therapy and Epilepsy

PENNY

Tall, willowy, model-thin Penny looked older than fourteen. She had fair luminous skin and bright blue eyes which, unlike the heavy, dreary look I had encountered in another epileptic, had a merry glint to them. They were remarkably expressive eyes, and I learned to use them as a kind of barometer of Penny's mercurial passions. In fact, she was so dynamically different from the dull, brain-damaged epileptic patients I had worked with at a state hospital, that I found it hard to accept the fact that Penny had been having petit and grand mal seizures since she was ten.

Penny walked into our first session about five minutes late, looking reluctant and literally dragging her stylish clogs along the floor. She was dressed in skintight jeans embroidered with flowers, a braless see-through shirt, and a wide leather belt which encircled her tiny waist. Superficially,

Penny seemed a thoroughly stereotyped teen-ager, though she was more seductive looking than most. Yet the tension of her body belied the sex-nymph image she tried to project. Her head jutted forward, and her neck strained turtle fashion between her raised shoulders. Her facial expression was somewhere between skepticism and annoyance. Penny stopped a few feet from the group and stood there, nervously tugging on her long, dark hair.

I held out my hand to her. "Won't you join us?" I asked.

Penny shrugged her shoulders. "Nah, you look like such assholes prancing around here. I don't know what the hell you're doing in this shitty place, anyway."

Twenty-four-year-old Don, who, along with the group, had been swinging the trunk of his body downward in a tension-free swaying motion, now raised his head to inspect the new patient. He seemed instantaneously smitten. The pupils of his eyes dilated, his nostrils quivered. Alert and interested, like a bird dog sniffing quail, Don left us to our tension-free swings and walked quickly over to Penny.

"You're right," he said. "It *is* crazy here." He ducked his head apologetically, "Except sometimes it's not sooooo bad!"

At that, Penny was all dimples and smiles. Her eyes sparkled. She leaned over and whispered something conspiratorially to Don, using her long hair as a screen. Don nodded his head and laughed. Through Penny's strands of wavy hair, Don flashed me a guilty look, but then quickly turned back to Penny. They lit cigarettes, and Don, his hand held gallantly under Penny's elbow, propelled her to the couch, where they proceeded to dismiss me and dance therapy from their minds.

I was prepared for this. I wanted to allow Penny this freedom of choice at least for her first few visits to the recreation room. Don was obviously enraptured and was aggressively taking his own brand of therapeutic enrichment. I was delighted, for I deemed his courtship of Penny more important than any tension-free swing, particularly when this was the first time in my memory that Don had seemed attracted to a girl. At twenty-four, he had had one homosexual encounter and had never been emotionally attached to any woman but his mother. I made a mental note to discuss Don's new interest further at the next staff meeting. I was particularly interested in finding out if the other therapists felt Don's attraction was due to the fact that he did not feel threatened by such a young girl.

I knew Penny would join the group eventually, but I wondered how long it would take her to capitulate. Watching her, I thought how difficult it must be for her to adjust herself to the sights and sounds of the recreation room. I hoped that Penny would adjust, since I felt that she could benefit from the therapeutic, cathartic bath that dance therapy could provide.

I hoped, too, that Penny would come to recognize the uniqueness of the dance therapy room. In a sense, it was a sanctuary. In dance therapy neither I nor my patients were concerned with practical matters such as bed-making, washing, eating, sleeping, cleaning, and basic hygiene, so that there was an undeniable, "honeymoon" quality about our sessions. Thus, while the live-in therapists had to be concerned with the patients' elementary functioning, I could luxuriate with the patients in a climate of sweet permissiveness. In fact, in order to achieve my goal of spontaneous movement, an air of freedom had to be established. In a sense, I was asking my patients to obey the rules outside of my province, and then walk through the portals of the recreation room and be free spirits. It was not always easy for some of them to do this. Dance therapy, as I structured it, was like having a favorite grandmother who felt you could do no wrong. You might have given your mother a hard time by not helping with the dishes, but your grandmother loved you simply because you existed.

Penny's reluctance to join the group reminded me of the behavior of an earlier patient at the clinic. Not that their pathology had been similar; she had not been a young epileptic, but a middle-aged professor of English, and a deeply depressed alcoholic. A highly articulate woman, she had never participated in sports or danced. Indeed, although her mouth went nonstop, she seemed to have no feeling for the rest of her body. She lumbered into every session on her two, stiff legs, her torso pitching forward in an unbroken line of tension. She would head for a chair in the corner where she would sit for the entire session, frowning and muttering, her back to the group.

Each week I would invite her to dance with us, stretching my arm out, palm upwards, in the "nonthreatening" gesture I had learned as a budding dance therapist. Invariably, she would turn her rigid body from me, mumbling her litany of hostility.

One day, after she had been with us for about two months, I happened to play Buddy Rich's drum solo record and suggested that we all vibrate our fingers and hands in response to the drumming. "Try working the vibration up through your arms—to your shoulders," I called out. "Now let your neck go—your head—your hips—your thighs—let your whole body vibrate!"

At long last our highly educated lady was titillated. Like the legendary phoenix rising from the ashes, she rose slowly from her chair and began tapping her foot.

"Are you doing the eighteenth-century Shaker movement?" she asked.

"You could call it that," I replied. "How about shaking the evil spirits out?" I asked.

She laughed. "God knows I need it," she said. "But actually, you're being rather simplistic, aren't you? There must have been deeply religious peaks of ecstasy for the Shaker performers, don't you agree?"

"You're right," I answered. I was determined to keep her up and moving as long as possible. "It must have been a cleansing, healing experience for many of them."

Though she looked annoyed, she kept jiggling. "I don't know how you can apply the principles of Shakerism in here," she said, describing the chaos of the room with a flourish of her hands. "We need more dignified surroundings to expound on the equality of the sexes, on efforts to avoid personal competition, and on the Shakers' love and respect for Nature."

I smiled. "That's a big order. But let's take them one at a time. How about vibrating for women's lib?"

The drums played on, as I watched our prolix patient respond to the beat. She began as I had suggested at her fingertips, and then proceeded to let what seemed to be an electric current of vibration run through her body until she was quivering and shaking in an emotional frenzy as authentic as any eighteenth-century Shaker. The rest of us, vibrating to a much lesser degree, were mesmerized by her dramatic movements. Finally, our "Shaker" fell to the floor, exhausted.

I put my arms around her, and in a moment or two she looked up at me.

"Words fail me," she said, grinning, "but, I think my consciousness has been raised!"

This patient took months to respond to the lure of dance therapy. Now I had another patient, Penny, who showed a similar avoidance of any conventional physical activity. Yet I knew by the flick of her hips when she walked that there was movement trapped in Penny's lithe, fourteen-year-old body.

In her fourth dance therapy session Penny stood apart, chain smoking and whispering behind her hand to anyone who would approach her.

Al Hirt's great trumpet solo of "I Can't Get Started With You," seared through the recreation room.

Penny stiffened. "Whaddaya know. My mother's favorite song."

"Is it?" I asked. "You know, it's a famous old blues classic."

The trumpet crying "I Can't Get Started," seemed quite descriptive of Penny's present condition. Her arms hung stiffly by her sides. Her head was pressed forward, putting her neck and back into constricted tension, so much that her shoulder blades stood out clearly, almost in a deformed way. Her long legs were stiff-kneed, one limb almost glued to the other. And yet oddly enough, there was movement in her hips as her body unconsciously reacted to the sound of Al Hirt's trumpet. There was a slight, insistent movement in her pelvis, forward and back, up and down. It was small, sexual, instinctive. But it was movement.

Penny quickly began to light another cigarette. I put my fingers lightly on her arm.

"Penny, my rule is no cigarettes while we're moving." Ignoring her scowl, I continued, "I have an idea. I'll bet you this record that I can make dance so absorbing for you that you won't feel the need for a cigarette. Will you try it?"

Penny's eyes bored into mine in the silence that followed. Carefully, she put the cigarette back in the pack.

"OK, I'll try. I'm trying to cut down anyway. Now what kind of friggin' stuff do you want me to do? That circle junk you do looks like my kid sister's 'ring around the rosie.'"

"I don't *want* you to do anything, Penny, except join us." Then I added, "*You* may want to do something then."

Penny's penetrating gaze moved around the circle, catching Brian in one of his mystical, godlike attitudes, his arms raised in benediction over Carol's head.

"So that's Jesus!" she whispered to me. "Do I really have to dance with these bananas?"

I put my hand lightly under her chin. "You could help them, and you might even learn from them."

Penny frowned. "OK. OK. But don't expect no miracles from me." She looked over at Brian, "I'll leave that to the messiah."

Penny took my outstretched hand, and we joined the others in the opening circle movement.

I grinned at Penny as she started to move her hips to the beat of the music. "Good girl! You're getting started."

Penny grinned back. "It's goddammed tough, though, you better believe it."

"Why so tough?" I asked.

"Oh, I don't know. I guess it's because I never know what people expect me to do," she said, moving her stomach muscles in and out, broadening her movement.

85

"It doesn't matter what anybody expects. What you're doing now is marvelous!"

Penny's cheeks flamed. "I don't know how *marvelous* it is. It's just a natural movement. I could always do this . . . and *this*, too!" At this, Penny triple-timed her pulsating stomach muscles, threw her arms out to the side, and spread her legs wide like a belly dancer.

Don, who was standing close to her, spoke in an awed whisper. "Hey, we got a go-go girl with us."

Penny giggled. "Boy, if I ever did this at home, my uncle would lay it on me. He says I'm a whore."

Suddenly, Penny's face clouded over. "I gotta stop. I'm dizzy," she said, her hand fluttering, her legs wobbly.

She did look shaken and pale, I thought, as I helped her over to the couch.

"Are you OK?" I asked, fearful that the dizzy spell might be a prelude to an epileptic attack.

"Yeah, I'm OK. Just kinda dizzy, and I feel sorta shaky inside, too."

I patted Penny's hand. "I think you'd better sit the rest out. Today was a great beginning. Let's put a bookmark in. We'll start next week where we left off."

Penny looked up at me wanly. "One thing . . . you were right. I didn't want a cigarette until just this moment. Do I still get the record if I smoke one now?"

"Absolutely. We honor bets in here, you know."

Penny took a deep drag and blew a smoke ring in my face. "You may run out of records before I run out of cigarettes," she said.

I laughed. "You're worth a whole stack of 'em."

As I packed my records away for the day, I mused about Penny. Could her dizziness have been triggered by the mention of her uncle? An experience that I had had some years before with an epileptic at the state hospital flashed through my mind. My patient there was a forty-eight-year-old woman whose seizures in dance therapy had been triggered by a song.

When I first beheld Mary at a dance therapy session, my eyes flew open unbelievingly. There she stood in the doorway, a heavy, shapeless body, a face bereft of expression, dreary eyes, with strands of lifeless red hair strewn about her face. Perched on her head was a bright blue football helmet. My first thought was that a patient scheduled for football practice had wandered into dance therapy by mistake. But there had been no error. The helmet was, in fact, a protection against skull concussions that might be incurred by this woman's frequent falls on the cement floor.

In reading the charts before our session, I had learned that Mary's forlorn condition reflected the extreme stresses of her life. She seemed to have lived totally without allies. Her mother, ashamed of her daughter's epilepsy, had abandoned her at thirteen. At seventeen, physically attractive despite her problems, she had married a volatile older man who beat her severely for her inadequacies. Later, her two teen-aged boys, who lacked adequate home supervision, established police records. By the time I met Mary, she had had sixty-three electric shock treatments.

Although my classes at the state hospital were large, I tried to give Mary some individual attention. She came willingly, loved music, and enjoyed being in charge of the record player. Her selection of records never varied—marches, folk music, and anything that I could bring her of Frank Sinatra. After a few weeks, I was fearful that we would have to drop dance therapy from Mary's program. Although she obviously enjoyed dancing, it was reported to me that her seizures occured more frequently in dance therapy than anywhere else. She fell backwards, forwards, and sidewards, indiscriminately, her only real pattern being that she landed with her legs slightly spread and with two fingers in her vagina.

Had it not been for an oversight on my part, I might never have recognized the stimulus for Mary's seizures. Hurrying to leave for the hospital one rainy morning, I left some of my record collection behind. Riffling through the stack, Mary was extremely disappointed.

"Boy, you really messed up this time, Mrs. Lefco. No Sinatra. No Frankie-boy. Jeez, I don't even feel like staying."

I put my arms around Mary's waist, and felt her wiggle furiously away from me. "I'm sorry about that, Mary. I'll remember to bring Frankie next week. But I do have some other records you might like—marches and a new Greek folk album. C'mon, be a good sport."

Mary turned her back to me hostilely, but nonetheless went over to the record player and put on the Greek record. Then we formed a circle and did some basic Greek dance movements. Mary held my hand and seemed interested in learning the steps. I showed her a fairly simple combination, which she enjoyed. We did some Greek feet-stomping, which seemed to release the anger she felt about being robbed of Frankie. Suddenly, after three-quarters of the session had gone by, I realized that Mary had had no seizures.

Checking her charts after the class had ended, I noted that her medication had not been changed in any way. In fact, the only difference in our program today had been the absence of the Frank Sinatra records. Could it be the famed Sinatra voice that caused Mary to have seizures?

Frank Sinatra was safely tucked under my arm when I arrived for my next session with Mary. This time, I handled the record player. First, I played marches. Mary joined in spiritedly, pumping her knees high in the air, working her arms like pistons, and inexpertly, but enthusiastically, twirling a baton which the hospital provided. She seemed in high spirits. Then I permitted the mellow sound of Sinatra to flood the room.

Mary beamed at me. "Wow, you remembered!" she said happily. "That boy sure gets to me." Mary's hips were now freely undulating, yet her trunk remained characteristically stiff, appearing almost divorced from the free, sensual action going on below. Her eyes were dreamy and somewhat glazed.

Yet after a few minutes of hip rolling, Mary suddenly made a small, animal sound and fell backward to the floor. She seemed dazed, but conscious, and I helped her to her feet and straightened her helmet. Though she was wobbly, she seemed ready to go on. As an experiment, I quickly changed the record to a quiet Strauss waltz. Hearing the music, Mary twirled around, sang a bit, moved her arms in a parody of a ballet dancer, and seemed calm and recovered.

For our last record of the session, I put Frankie on. Mary promptly had another seizure.

For the next few sessions I played Sinatra in small doses. As soon as I heard the first small, animal sound coming from Mary's lips, I quickly put my arms around her.

"Hold on, Mary. Stay with Frankie-boy. Don't leave him now." My first ministrations were a disaster. In spite of my voiced suggestions and comforting arms, Mary fell to the floor. After a few weeks, however, she was able to catch herself at the first sound of her characteristic moan. She would consciously snap her head back in position, and almost mechanically continue her hip rolls. Brain-damaged, beaten by life, Mary nonetheless seemed to be responding to large-muscle movements, to love, to arms around her, to a friend, to the physical closeness of another person. She still had petit and grand mal seizures outside of dance therapy, but at least in one area I had succeeded in relating Mary's seizures with her powerful, but inhibited, sexual response to Sinatra.

When I left the hospital at the end of a year, Mary was dancing through an entire Sinatra record without a seizure. Furthermore, she was doing it joyfully, healthfully, her body no longer at odds with itself, but moving in one coordinated movement.

Could this technique work for an epileptic like Penny, who was younger and whose symptoms in dance therapy had progressed no further than dizziness? I felt that she could be helped.

Realizing that I needed more information on Penny's relationship with her uncle, I headed for the office. Here, in the repository of coffee machines, typewriters, secretaries, time sheets, and case histories, I settled back to read Penny's reports from the therapist assigned to her case and from the social worker who was directly involved with the family. Two paragraphs interested me particularly:

Penny comes to us as a runaway, after being released from the police after her last flight from home. She was recovered after having a sexual relationship with a sixteen-year-old boy. Both of them were high on marijuana. They also admitted to having a few bourbons. Penny admits that she knows alcohol could be fatal to her when on her present medication. This fourteen-year-old epileptic girl has been running away from home since the age of 11, because it is "shitty" at home. She states that she hates her uncle, her divorced mother's brother who lives with them.

(Written by the social worker)

Penny seems to work under the assumption that if she is loved, she must be loved at her worst. She calls her younger brother a "goody-goody" and is striving for equal love from her mother. Penny feels that her mother is disappointed because her epilepsy makes her less perfect. Penny voluntarily denied any sexual feelings toward her uncle, but since she initiated the subject, there may be some deep feelings within her.

(Written by the therapist)

I chewed my lower lip thoughtfully. If, in dance therapy, we could act out some of Penny's sexual feelings toward her uncle; if I could illuminate for Penny the naiveté of her sexual fantasies; and if I could put her into a physically trusting situation with another male, possibly Don, she might abandon her seductive behavior and enjoy a wholesome relationship with someone of the opposite sex.

If I could ... but I couldn't! Had I a log of controlled experiments with epileptics, I might have attempted to go further into behavioral techniques applied to epileptics in dance therapy sessions. But since my experience had been limited to a handful of epileptic patients, I was not ready to deal with a technique that, if handled inexpertly, might endanger the very spontaneity that I sought to release. It was important to me that I concentrate on what I had found to be effective for neurotics, psychotics, epileptics, the labeled and the unlabeled; indeed, all people who were simply not at ease with their body's responses.

Keeping these ideas in mind, I began planning how I would augment Penny's physical movements, making them not only larger, but more forceful. I wanted each gesture to be a healthy, direct channeling of Penny's surplus electrical energy. From my reading, I had learned to differentiate movements into "clonic" and "tonic" categories. Clonic movements were almost like the movements of an epileptic seizure: abrupt, inconclusive, scattered. Contrarily, tonic gestures were strong, healthy, natural, conclusive, with a sequential message to the brain. Hopefully, I could lead Penny into tonic movements, which would provide healthy outlets for the discharge of her energy.

From further information gleaned at staff meetings, I learned of Penny's habitual refusal to "put herself on the line" for fear of failure. In all facets of her life at the clinic, she needed total acceptance before she would make the first move. Here, I felt, dance therapy could help. By using a technique of gentle persuasion, acceptance, praise, and encouragement for the slightest physical accomplishment, I felt that we could restore some confidence in Penny.

From our first dance therapy session, I realized that Penny was testing me. Her sulky demeanor and her foul language were calculated to provoke me and to demand my attention through her bad behavior. As often as I could, I gave her what she needed, my undivided attention with one-to-one intensity. Unfortunately, other patients, too, had their needs, and it was when I turned from her, that Penny would storm off, grab a cigarette, and stand belligerently on the fringe of the group.

However, as time progressed, I came to admire Penny's control, though in a larger sense, that very control might prove unhealthy since she tended to turn her anger inward. Although she might have run away easily from the recreation room, she remained, sometimes joining in, more often standing apart. But frightened, angry, uncertain as she was, she stayed with me. In essence, she wanted to please me, and she wanted me to praise her, to love her. When she began to allow herself to feel how much I cared, her movements, like the petals of a rose, unfolded, expanded, blossomed.

One day I discovered an old polka record at the clinic, and I put it on the record player. Penny much preferred contemporary rock to any other music, but I felt that while she had made much progress using her arms and her trunk, her legs were still held tensely and the polka rhythm might induce some large-muscle leg action. Turning from the record player, I braced myself for the hoots that I knew would greet the opening bars of the polka, for this sprightly dance seemed headed for extinction with the young folk. Yet knowing of Penny's Polish heritage, I hoped that the sound and beat of the polka might awaken an early memory for her.

"Aw, for shit's sake," Carol said, snapping her long hair around, exhibiting her characteristic low tolerance for frustration. "Do we have to go through this ethnic crap? Hey, Mrs. Lefco, why not tell a few Polack jokes while you're at it?" Carol warmed to the task, and the impish expression on her face made her look years younger than her actual twenty. "Did you hear the one about the Polack who hijacked a submarine? He wanted three thousand dollars and two parachutes."

"Shut up," Penny said, two spots of color appearing on her cheekbones. "You know my uncle's Polish."

"Oh for Christ's sake," Carol said. "Nothing personal, Penny." Carol grinned and held out her hand. "You don't really think I'm a goddammed bigot, do you?"

Penny smiled back. "Nah, forget it. I guess I'm sort of sensitive about those corny jokes, that's all."

"Have you ever danced any polkas, Penny?" I asked.

Penny threw her hands in front of her face. "Nope, Not me. Don't look at me for that stuff!" She then added wistfully, "My mother does the polka though, with my uncle. They like to horse around a lot."

The bouncy, polka rhythm filled the room. Almost as though I had arranged it, Don approached Penny in an old-fashioned, formal manner, as if he had his cap in his hand.

"May I have this dance, Penny?"

Penny was embarrassed. She shook her head.

"C'mon, Penny, it's fun," Don coaxed.

Impulsively, Penny responded in a parody of nineteenth-century dance etiquette formality. Stretching both arms toward Don, she threw back her head, exposing her long pale neck.

"I accept your offer to dance," she said suddenly.

Don took her extended hands, as he cocked his blond head to one side to observe her beauty. For a moment Don and Penny stood poised like two long-throated herons about to begin a ritualistic mating dance. And then they were off, their faces lit with merriment, their feet taking giant, awkward strides which seemed to propel their bodies into the air and down again with a clatter. Unconcerned with conventional footwork, their exuberance was uncontained and they danced around the room for a full five minutes.

"That's some stupid polka!" Carol called out from her prone position on the couch. "And you two look pretty damn stupid doing it!"

Her comment had the effect of a gunshot. Penny instantly stopped dancing, and looked down at her feet in confusion. When she looked up again, there were tears in her eyes.

"I told you I couldn't do this friggin' thing," she yelled at me. She put her hands to her temples. "I feel lousy. I want a cigarette."

Quickly, like a circus master, I began moving, shouting, directing traffic.

"Wait up. Hold it everyone. Penny, the polka isn't stupid, and you didn't look stupid. It was positively great, unique, creative. Where is it written that you have to polka a certain way?"

"Forget it," Penny said, her hand to her pale cheek. "I wanna sit down."

"Before you sit down, I want to show you something that will make you feel better," I said.

"Oh God, Mrs. Lefco, will you just let me sit down? I think I'm gonna conk out." Two tears rolled down her cheeks as she nervously fingered her pants pocket, searching for her cigarettes."

I took Penny's hand in mine. "I won't let you fall. Trust me."

Penny's breathing was shallow. Her normally bright blue eyes looked darker and duller. "What now?"

"First take some deep breaths. I'll count to five while you inhale. Now see that your stomach gets fat . . . and then I'll count another five while you exhale . . . and see how skinny your tummy gets. Start now."

It was a great effort for Penny to comply. She was pale and trembling, and it took physical courage and faith for her to stand her ground. She took a deep breath in and out. As I nodded encouragement, she took another slow, protracted breath and exhaled. She held up a finger.

"Lemme try one more," she said.

After three deep yoga breaths, the color returned to Penny's cheeks. She was now breathing normally. I squeezed her hand. "Good girl. Sit down now for a minute, and then let's you and me do the wildest polka anyone's ever seen."

Penny laughed and the corners of her mouth turned way up. "You are the living end," she said, and then whispered in my ear, "witch doctor."

As Penny rested, I was free to turn my attention to the group. "OK, kids, as long as Carol thinks Penny and Don were doing a stupid polka, let's really scrap the rule book and do a whole new thing. Everybody grab a partner! We are now going to attempt for the first time in the center ring, the ultramad, way-out, something else, 'back-to-back' polka. C'mon, Penny, are you ready now?"

Penny nodded and stood up with no trace of shakiness or hesitancy.

Carol lowered her eyes, quietly. She had heard her word "stupid" mirrored and recognized how destructive it had been to Penny. She sprang from the couch saying, "Penny, may I do the 'back-to-back' polka with you?"

Penny giggled, her blue eyes once again bright and alert. "Sure," she said. "But first," and she turned to Don, "watch how the experts do it."

The group watched as Don and Penny turned their backs to one another and stretched their arms out, clasping their hands tightly together. Their heads touched, and their cheeks turned toward each other, as they both smiled triumphantly. Penny sighed deeply. Her back was pressed firmly against Don, her shoulder blades flat against his back. Her chest rose, her head lifted. She seemed to be luxuriating in the closeness and warmth of her partner, and in the support he provided for her in this position.

Penny wiggled and flexed her back muscles against Don's back. "Ooooooh, this feels good," she said. "Wow! a human back rub. Look ma! No hands!"

Don, too, seemed at ease with the arrangement. He stretched and arched and rubbed his back against Penny's. "Hey, try it, you'll like it. Try it, Mrs. L." Don's eyes found mine. "This stuff is better than dancing any day."

"So who needs to dance?" Carol said, watching them closely. "You kids look good together, so stay the way you are. She turned to Brian, "Hey, lover, gimme a hunk of back. Let's do Penny's 'pooped-out polka!'" Carol winked over at Penny. "No offense, kids."

Our session ended with everyone trying the "pooped-out" polka. When Penny and Don finally did pull apart, Penny's back was straight, and she held her head erectly between her relaxed shoulders.

"How about this, Mrs. L.?" she said, lighting a cigarette. "It's my first drag since I walked in. Think I'm gonna make it?"

I smacked her gently on her little rump. "I know you're going to make it. My money's on you, Penny."

Though she was almost out the door, she suddenly turned back, ran over to me, kissed me lightly on the cheek, and then bolted from the room.

Whether that kiss was just teen-age exuberance, or whether it was for the physical release that she experienced by dancing the polka, for the yoga breathing that had pulled her back from the edge of an epileptic attack, or possibly for the support she received from me after Carol's attack—I'll never know.

CHAPTER VII

We Dance a Dream

DON

I am always eager to attend a staff meeting, where the stimulus of the staff's original, open-minded thinking far outweighs the discomfort of the small room in which we meet. Our meeting room is located in the main building, a white, heavily decorated Victorian relic, which sits front and center of our compound. The image of this old, gingerbread edifice facing a cement driveway filled with new Volkswagon campers underscores our philosophy at the Institute. We are all irrefutably linked to our past.

Staff members convene here once a week, bringing their youth, their vitality, and their individualism through the narrow doors. An inadequate cluster of hard, straight chairs and small couches forces most of the therapists to sit cross-legged on the floor, an informality that belies the intensity of the life-and-death decisions made here. Sprawled on the fraying carpet and slumped against the walls are approximately twenty to thirty staff members—the director, family therapists, clinical psychologists, psychiatrists, undergraduate students interning at the clinic, and ancillary therapists of music, art, dance, and drama.

There are thin, Christlike figures in faded blue jeans who finger their beards and pull thoughtfully at their mustaches. There are young women in African-print cotton dresses and bare feet, while others wear no-nonsense skirts and sweaters. There is a sprinkling of cowboy boots and Navajo silver jewelry, as well as an Establishment business suit. "If it is comfortable for you, we're happy" could be the slogan here.

Sitting in the center of the room, swiveling around in a high-backed, nineteenth century office chair, is the medical director. Over his head hangs a large poster of a woman's face, a grim, humorless, lantern-jawed female, wearing a small black hat jammed down on her forehead. Written under the poster are the sentences, "Talk to me. I am your mother."

Indeed, there is a certain irony to this juxtaposition of the director and "mother," for the director stresses that some patients attribute their cure to finding a "mother" in him. He is the mother they never had in actuality, the mother most closely allied to the image in each patient's heart. I know that in my own experience with patients in dance therapy, the mention of the word "mother" always elicits a dramatic body reaction—fists clench, mouths tighten, eyes blaze, shoulders sag. It seems that none of the patients feel that their mothers lived up to the ideal, which is surely one reason why they are here.

At one o'clock, an anticipatory hush falls over the room, and the meeting begins. Prosaic clinic problems are first on the agenda to be discussed. There are broken drains to be fixed, plans for a new building, and the mystifying disappearance of bed linen from the supply closet. The question always at the forefront is the knotty one of who will clean the recreation room. Traditionally, the family unit—two therapists and their three patients—are assigned to cleanups, but the unit results are invariably uneven. Invidious allegations begin to fly back and forth. One family with a strong cleaning record feels they are being undermined by a slovenly unit. The art therapist and I cry out our grievances, too. Forced to work on a floor strewn with cigarette butts, pieces of clay, and kitty litter, we bitterly resent past, unkept promises. The entire second floor rings with vigorous assaults and rebuttals, and finally, subdued compromises.

With this out of our systems, we are ready to proceed to the heart of the meeting—a discussion of psychiatric techniques and theories, a progress report on a special case, or a detailed background of a new patient. With each subject comes the additional stimulus of open discussion between the therapists and the medical director. Since all of us have spent considerable time with mental patients and have seen the pathetic results of lives crippled by lies and deceptions, we have learned to be bluntly honest with ourselves and with others. Staff meetings can be shocking to the uninitiated, for the amenities of the socialized world are often ignored, and superficial charm is in short supply.

Today, the medical director is airing a critical case which requires immediate attention from all staff members. Following a visit from his father, and a jolting letter from his mother, Don has tried to hang himself.

Don is twenty-four-years old and has been at the clinic for five years. Prior to this, he had been in another mental hospital for two years. Wafer-thin, but a handsome lad by any standards, Don has a high round forehead, fine, long blond hair, light eyes set wide apart, and a nose and mouth of movie star proportions. Don manages to keep these good looks well-hidden, however, for he carries his head forward of his body, where it hangs like the head of a whipped hound dog, eyes down, mouth drooping. He is the product of an authoritarian father who himself had inherited from his family the notion that there should be only one voice in the family, the father's. Don's mother, passive, frightened, devious, had turned to religion. Yet she had not yet given up on saving her son through religion since she believed that demons were inhabiting him.

Don's father had left home when Don was sixteen. "Even that was long overdue," he had said, according to the inky-bearded therapist who reported the conversation to us. "He said," the therapist added, "that there was nothing left in that house. His wife was a religious fanatic, and Don was nuts . . . and half a pansy to boot. The only pleasure he got was from his youngest son, who was like him and could take care of himself. He's convinced that his wife will probably make the second son crazy too."

"I'd like to read a part of the letter Don just received from his mother," continued the therapist. He shook his massive head of black curls in dismay. "No wonder the poor bastard is so confused."

We all listened with interest.

"'. . . and, of course, we all want you to be at your brother's investiture. I will be so proud of you because you will be the best-looking man there. You really belong with your family. Try to come.'"

We Dance a Dream

As he read these last words Don's therapist tugged tensely at his beard. "Christ! Don received the letter three days *after* the ceremony took place!"

We all winced at the thought of Don's mother's empty invitation.

"He didn't say much about the letter," the therapist continued, looking up wryly. "He didn't have to. Talk about body action, Helene," he said in my direction. "Even without your training you could see despair in the way he's been skulking around. And this letter on top of a rough visit from his old man when he threatened to yank Don out of the clinic again. Wow!" he added, "you don't have to be crazy to snap."

"True," intervened the medical director, "but Don *is* crazy, and since he did try to commit suicide three days ago, I still want him watched around the clock—twenty-four-hour surveillance—sleeping, eating, defecating."

"Oh—defecating—that reminds me," said the lovely Spanish wife of the curly haired therapist. "Maybe this should have come up earlier, with the clinic problems, because in essence, it's a plumber's problem. Don keeps stuffing up the toilets. And for Pete's sake, he only uses them half as much as anyone else!"

"Say, maybe we could get him his own potty," the art therapist suggested. "Could be he wants to play with his feces. He probably never had a chance to. You know, in my class, Don loves playing with wet clay. I've got some samples of his work here in my bag. Would you like to see them?"

We all nodded, since most of us had seen some revealing art work originate from the unprepossessing corner of the recreation room, known as the art therapy shop.

The art therapist dived into an enormous brown envelope where she kept samples of her patients' work. Finding a piece of Don's clay sculpture, she passed it around the room.

"Hey," the music therapist called out, fingering Don's handiwork, "this is the first bit of art therapy work that I can interpret unequivocally." She looked around at us all with a grin. "Am I being overly simplistic, or is this actually a piece of shit?"

All the talk of primitive bowel functioning reminded me of the book, *Mary Barnes: Two Accounts of a Journey Through Madness,* by Mary Barnes and Dr. Joseph Berke [New York: Harcourt Brace Jovanovich, Inc., 1972]. It is the tale of a young mental patient in East London who was encouraged by her doctor to paint pictures on the wall with her feces as one phase of her cure. I wondered whether our clinic was geared to handle such protracted regression. But, techniques aside, I hoped that we could work with Don so that he, like Mary Barnes would say of the clinic, "It is a place to go down, and come back."

A vision of Don as I knew him in dance therapy popped into my head. I saw his tense solar plexus and the tautness of his entire body. During the first year of our sessions, his ability to express joy, grief, or anger was so minimal that if I weren't watching closely, I would miss the movement entirely. He was doubtless as loath to part with his feces as he was to make any revealing gesture. How desperately he seemed to withhold his rage, his anger, his frustration. The only explosive release he permitted himself was the letting go of his bowels and urine. Even there, he was afraid of the release, so much so that when he did use the toilet, he stuffed it with toilet paper to prevent a part of him from being flushed away.

During Don's first months at the clinic, he skulked around like Frankenstein, in and out of dance therapy. Head down, bent arms held up high, hands drooping at the wrists, Don let his body shuffle along. He had come from another institution where he had been heavily tranquilized, and where he had received twenty electric shock treatments. Don had been treated for his drug habits—marijuana, hashish, amphetamines—and was eventually cured of his addiction. Don's real problems surfaced only after he came to our clinic. Here he wet the bed nightly. During the day he soiled his pants. He was in turn sepulchrally quiet, or noisily hostile. Sometimes he could be murderously angry, shouting and cursing and screaming like a maddened religious zealot. Spent, he would settle back in a passive mood for months at a time. After a visit from either of his parents, Don would be deeply depressed. Then the whole bizarre cycle, starting with the monster walk, would begin again.

Don's attempted suicide this time was an entirely new development. He had changed his pattern. The medical director felt that, in a perverse way, Don was beginning to get well. Even his attempted suicide could be interpreted as a "healthy" sign, odd terminology for such a tragic act. But perhaps it was healthy in that at long last, Don was beginning to get in touch with his anger, no longer disguising it from himself with his myriad forms of bizarre emotional armoring.

Throughout five years of dance therapy with Don, I tried to encourage him to relax his guard, loosen up physically, and express his anger. He was fearful of women, and therefore especially distrustful of me, because our sessions always involved touching and body awareness. Don tensed and con-tracted with anxiety whenever he had to react with his body. I could only touch him if he reached for my hand, which was a rare occurrence.

Generally, Don preferred to do a little "dance" alone, far away from the circle of patients, secreted deep in a corner. As soon as the music began, and any music would do for Don, he would hang his head even lower than usual, bend his knees, crumple his midsection, and hang limply forward like a tired kangaroo, while he gently swayed to the rhythm. When the beat quickened, he would lift one leg from the floor, and then put it down woodenly. Then he would lift the other leg. His pale blond hair fell over his face, as he breathed deeply and evenly. When the record finished, he would lift his head high, look around him in wonderment, and smile. "Boy, that was fun," he said invariably.

If I tried to intrude by swinging along with him, he would discontinue all movement. If I talked to him, questioned him, or even came into his field of vision, he would walk away. Don wanted to do this dance himself, in his own way, and I permitted him this freedom. For a long time, dance therapy meant little more to Don than his kangaroo swing in the corner. But the refreshed look on his face when he finished his dance seemed to signify that he was getting what he needed.

In Don's fourth year at the clinic, he met a new patient, Penny, fourteen and chock-full of precocious sex appeal. She had come into dance therapy, swinging her hips, and, as the kids say, "the vibes were good." Amazingly, Don maneu-vered himself close to her. For the first time, he joined the circle formation when Penny held out her hand to him. Don's feelings of excitement were reflected in his eyes and in his face as he shyly took her hand. My God! He is overwhelmingly smitten, I thought, and hallelujah, he's not fighting it!

Don's therapist's voice suddenly snapped me back to the staff meeting.

"Don keeps having this recurrent dream," the curly haired therapist was saying. "It seems that he's in a swimming meet, along with his brother. The coach calls out, 'On your mark. Go!' Everyone dives in, and Don is leading the pack. Suddenly two voices are shouting to him from the stands. He stops swimming and tries to make out what they're saying as all the swimmers pass him.

"I've heard him sobbing during the night," he continued, "and when I get to him, he's got a load in his pants. Yet nothing that I've said to him so far has stopped the dream from recurring. Anybody got any ideas?"

For a few minutes we listened to the dream interpretations put forth by the various staff members.

A deep voice rumbled up from the floor. It came from a tall young man, a psychologist, who had part of his chestnut mane pulled back in a ponytail and the rest held in place by a beaded Indian headband. As he sat sprawled on the floor, his tremendously long legs suggested the professional basketball career that he had before joining the clinic. An avowed follower of the Gestalt technique, the psychologist strongly advocated the theory that the body must physically permit feelings to rise to the surface.

"Say, why don't you try dancing the dream, Helene?" he asked me. "Maybe Don would level with himself if he could relive the dream—act it out—in your workshop. I mean, maybe the physical approach should be explored. God knows what we've done so far hasn't worked!"

The psychologist's words stuck in my mind, and I must confess that I heard very little more of the concluding parts of the staff meeting.

To dance a dream? To dance a dream . . . not as a ballet, not as a Shakespearean fantasy, but as a simple story with moving parts. Perhaps even a small segment of the swimming dream could be transformed into a piece of pantomime, where body movement and body reactions might bring insight to Don.

Although I had never "danced a dream" before, nor had I heard of any dance therapist who had "dream-danced," I had read extensively on the subject of dreams. While I was an admirer of the Freudian interpretation for the consultation room, for the dance therapy session I thought I would be more comfortable with Jung, for he concentrated on the content of a dream and what it might reveal, rather than what it might conceal. I warmed to the whole idea when I remembered the words of our medical director, "If it works, it's a good technique."

Don *could* dance his dream. But *would* he?

The next day, a blustery morning when we were almost barricaded in the recreation room by mounds of snow, I stomped in to work. Fortunately the winter season was in my favor, for the weather is an influential factor in the recreation room. Here inadequate weather stripping on all apertures gives the room the same reflection of nature that the Gurus find so appealing in the caves of the Himalayas. In the summer, without benefit of air-conditioning, with doors hanging open on rusty hinges, with window screens torn, the patients mope and sigh in the simmering heat. Large-scale movements are forsaken, and the emphasis is on light touching, cradling, and a gentle rock to soft music. In the winter, we are driven to keep moving to ward off the cold. Because doors are constantly opened by the continual in-and-out flow of patients and therapists, the arctic air of January blows in frequent gusts through the room. Although we have a heating system, the freezing drafts seem to predominate over the warmth. Today, with the temperature a low eighteen degrees outside, and only a bit higher inside, I planned to start the session early, if only to keep the dance therapist warm.

As I bravely took off my coat, I observed my patients in their usual stances of hostility. Some were leaning against posts, some slumped on couches, a few were standing stiffly in the center of the room waiting for something to happen. Defiance and indifference rather than fashion and the frigid temperature seemed to have designed their outfits. Don was wearing a white undershirt and Bermuda shorts. At first glance, Laura seemed appropriately dressed with a wool scarf around her neck and a heavy cap pulled over her forehead. But on closer inspection, I noticed that her legs were bare. Kevin was wearing his winter outfit, a Navy pilot's fleece-lined leather jacket, which I knew from experience that he would never remove, no matter how warm he got. Penny's tight cotton halter, postage-stamp mini-skirt, and bare midriff showed her defiance of convention and the freezing weather outside.

Anxious to get everyone moving quickly, I put on a record that was a group favorite, Elton John's "Honky Chateau," a beautiful sound of piano, bass, mandolin, and guitar.

In relation to the apathetic picture I had viewed minutes before, the music brought an almost immediate physical change in the scene.

"Wow. What a groovy sound. Fantastic!" Penny said, moving her arms in a wide arc and letting her pelvis swing freely back and forth, as her mini-skirt waved and swished around her bare thighs.

At the first chord, Brian began an awkward leap through space, circling the room with the ascendant speed of a cheetah, if not its coordinated grace.

All around me, I beheld movement, heads thrown back, shoulders lifting and lowering to the beat. I noticed too, with supreme satisfaction, that those who had been smoking cigarettes were stubbing them out. My patients know that I disapprove of smoking during a dance therapy session, and astonishingly enough, everyone is usually cooperative. Perhaps they are usually compliant because it is the only rule that I have laid out for them, or perhaps because I am substituting something with fresh appeal.

Don stood alone silently near the open door, almost motionless, his arms hanging dispiritedly by his side.

"Hey, Don," I asked, "would you mind closing the door? It seems to be snowing in here."

There was no answer. Don did not seem to realize that I had spoken.

"Don? Did you hear me? How about closing the door?"

Still no response! Suddenly, Penny flounced by me. "Fuh shit's sake, Don, are you so fucking paralyzed that you can't even close a simple door?"

Penny slammed the door, glaring furiously at Don. "God, you're crazy today," she said.

At that, there was a visible widening of Don's nostrils. He raised his head, opened his eyes wide, and stared at Penny.

"Bitch," he said.

Penny laughed and danced back to the center of the room, rolling her hips and gesturing obscenely with her finger in Don's direction.

I reached toward Don with my arm, and when he jerked his body away, I left the group and walked to his side.

"Don," I said quietly, "you seem to feel lousy today. Maybe, if you move, it will help."

Don shook his head. There were tears in his eyes. "Just bug off, will you?"

"Don," I said, the palm of my hand outstretched to him, "won't you try?"

With an enraged turn of his head, Don spit at me. For a minute we both stared at the spittle in the palm of my hand. When I looked up and our eyes met, Don's face seemed curiously free of tension.

"Feel better now?" I asked calmly.

Don hung his head with the embarrassment of a small boy caught in a mischievous act. "I'm sorry," he muttered. Then, unexpectedly, putting his palm on mine, he wiped up the little puddle, holding the contact of the palms of our hands for a long time.

"Hey, Don," Penny called, "c'mon over. We need you."

"I just want to watch for a while," Don said. "I wanna smoke this," he added, lighting a cigarette.

"OK, Don," I said, "but I'll be waiting for you when you finish."

The sound of Elton John, raised to full volume by Carol, filled the room. Penny and Carol were facing one another,

111

gyrating with the joyous unrestrained movements of "go-go" girls. They seemed to be vying for supremacy in a contest of muscular flexibility of the pelvis. Together, they had a power and thrust that was awesome, and the men in the group looked more than a bit threatened by this show of strength; they visibly backed off to give the girls room for their performance. Brian moved away, half-closing his eyes and holding onto his penis fearfully.

But Don was oblivious. When he finished his cigarette, he came shyly forward as he had promised. Then, mimicking the girls, he pawed the air, shaking his body convulsively, the way a dog might after being out in the rain. His hands flopped feebly around him, and he used the same narrow, physical vocabulary that characterized most of his movements.

"Make it larger, Don," I suggested. "Make everything stronger. Really push your way through the air like the postman had to do with the snow this morning to bring us our mail."

Don stiffened. I had touched a nerve. But I really hadn't meant to upset him by alluding to his mother's letter so early in the session. It had been on my mind, and more human being than therapist, the words were out of my mouth before I knew it.

"I don't want any goddamned letter," Don said.

"Show me with your body how you really feel when you don't want that letter," I said.

For a moment Don hesitated, looking wistfully toward the open door. But something made him change his mind, and he began slicing through the air, slashing his arms through space, his teeth gritted, his face red.

"Fuckin' letter!" he gasped.

"Hey, everybody," I called out, "let's make the postman take back the goddamn letter. Let's help Don get rid of that lousy letter he got from his mother!"

"Hah, that's easy!" Carol said. "You should see the shitty one I got from my old lady."

The group moved sympathetically toward Don, leaving their accustomed spots on the floor. I watched as shoulders moved aggressively, as chins angled pugnaciously. The group began, each in his or her own individual way, to push with hips, buttocks, elbows, the palms of their hands. They smacked and slapped and shoved one another, caught up in this fight against the hurting words of a letter. Don, concentrating on his own motions, seemed to be gathering momentum, as his arms pinwheeled about him. Forgetting the others for a moment, I concentrated on his movements and his rhythms. For a moment or two I pinwheeled in unison with Don, miming his every motion. We were actually stroking together like competitive Olympic swimmers. The moment I had been seeking to recreate had arrived unexpectedly. We were ready to help Don relive his dream.

"Where are we?" I asked.

"In a pool."

"Where?"

"In the school swimming pool," Don said. Then it clicked in his brain. "I had a dream like this."

"Who's in the pool with you?"

"My brother."

"Anybody else around?"

"Yeah, some big broad in the stands with her husband."

The rest of the patients had stopped moving when I shifted my attention to Don. I turned to them now. "Hey, we're in a swimming meet with Don. How about jumping into the pool with us?"

Brian, always fey, attempted to do a back dive. Carol gracefully set herself the task of a swan dive.

"Here I come," screeched Penny, giggling as she followed her outstretched arms headlong to the floor.

Laura jumped in next, fingers pinching her nostrils. Kevin was dog-paddling. Now we were all in the water together.

Don was still frantically pinwheeling his arms. Carol, beside him, was competitively stretching out beyond him.

"I'll beat you, you sonovabitch," she said.

"C'mon you faggot, move!" The voice was Brian's, and the words were those that I had heard many times before. A master at projecting his feelings, Brian blasted many of the male patients with the fury he felt for himself. But this time his voice and his words fit perfectly into Don's dream. It might easily have been the voice of his father in the stands.

Reacting immediately to Brian's outburst, Don stopped moving. His pants suddenly darkened. He stood very still, his head sunk to his breast as a strong odor filled the room.

"Phew! Wotta stink!" Carol said. "Everybody outa the pool. Someone's crapped in it!"

I put my hand comfortingly on Don's shoulder, even though I was uncontrollably gagging at the strong odor.

"Get your lousy hands off me," he snarled. "I'm sick to death of you and your voice."

"Did you hear my voice?" I managed to say, backing off a bit.

"You're goddamn right, I did," Don said. "I heard you and the old man screaming for my brother to win."

"Not me, Don," I said. "I've always rooted for you."

"And them? What about them? What were they screaming about?"

"What do you think?" I asked.

"I don't know . . . I don't know . . . ," Don's voice trailed off. Then he looked down at his stained pants and mumbled ". . . but it scares the shit out of me every time."

As the session ended and the patients left the room, I again recalled the director's words, "If it works, it's a good technique."

Had it worked? There was no doubt that Don *had* relived a haunting experience, and that a large amount of tension had been relieved. But for him to resolve his torment he would need continued help from all quarters. Perhaps, in our next few sessions, he could be encouraged to repeat the release he had achieved today. A recurring dream might well require recurring physical treatments.

Under a cold, clean, noonday sky, I headed briskly toward the office typewriter to write my report on how Don had danced his dream.

CHAPTER VIII

Pencil and Paper Approaches

Several weeks later, at the end of a particularly exhilarating, exhausting session, Don walked over to me and quietly slipped a small piece of paper into the back pocket of my jeans.

Dear Mrs. L.,
Dance therapy is better than a straitjacket.

Don

I smiled as I deciphered the light, cramped, fuzzy handscript, but then I recalled my annoyance the week before when Don had appeared for dance therapy encumbered by a straitjacket. I had immediately scribbled a note to his therapist, requesting permission to remove the jacket for our next session. I added that I would accept full responsibility for Don, to see that he neither ran off, nor did damage to himself or to others. It was not as tall an order as it sounded, since I knew by experience that Don had a penchant for "dancing out" his frustrations in our sessions. The family therapist had granted my request, and, judging from the note, Don had profited by the experience of being free and unfettered during dance therapy.

Later, thinking about Don's note, I wondered if I could prod my other patients to *write* what they would or could not *say.* I wondered, too, if patients who were tense and "frozen" physically could be helped to communicate in this manner, and so I began to elicit written responses to my queries.

I tried distributing paper and pens in our last five minutes of a session, and asked each patient to answer one general question about the dance therapy session he had just experienced. Sometimes I had the patients describe their moods on paper twice, both at the beginning and at the end of a session. They did not have to identify themselves if they preferred anonymity. But some were happy to see themselves identified by name on a page.

My results showed me some of the nontalkers, as well as some of the "mixed-salad" or bumbling talkers, can be both prolific and lucid on paper. Over a period of a few months I collected more revealing, apt, and downright funny critiques and comments than I believed were possible. The following are representative of the hundreds of responses I received:
What part of you feels the best after dance therapy?
    "My penis. Is that what you want me to say?"
    "My toes. My clothes."
    "All but my neck."

118

"My bottom."

"My legs feel loose."

"My whole body feels sexcited . . . and good, too."

"The music, the beat, and my body became one, and for a few minutes I am very much alive."

How did dance therapy help you today?

"Helped?"

"It made me happy and limber. Ready for action."

"Dance is great. Better than sleep."

"My back hurt and now it doesn't."

"I moved my body in directions which seemed weird."

"At first I felt constricted, dead. After dancing for a while I enjoyed the tired sweatiness, enjoyed feeling my own body more relaxed, more in touch with myself. . . . I liked watching Helene work with Kevin to make him move. But after being here I'm aware of a certain sadness in myself that I can't figure out. . . ."

"It didn't help me. I was worried when I came in and I'm still worried. I want to rot. Just rot. And you, you are the weirdest dancing teacher I ever saw."

"This is the first time I liked dance therapy. It stank last week. This week it was more informal and everyone could move the way they wanted. I was glad that I refused to join the circle. I didn't want to touch anyone today."

How do you feel after dance therapy today?

"I feel sorry for you. You sure need 'balls' to take this job!"

"Tired, with a feeling of healthiness, meaning something constructive. Loose . . .arms, legs, hips, etc."

"I'd like my legs to be hotter. They're still cold."

"My arms expressed a lot for me today."

"The body is the way things are . . .ha, ha, ha."

"I feel tired, rundown, and unhappy. I need pills."

"I would say dominant, cuddled, and loose."

"I noticed that I dance backward—like I do everything else. I guess that means I'm afraid."

What does dance therapy do for you?

"It makes me know that *more and more attention must be paid.*"

"I really like the dancing and look forward to it. It has helped me with body awareness and to become 'looser.' I always disliked dancing. I do not feel that way at dance therapy. Some of the people sit around sometimes and do not participate. This gives me more attention, but it sometimes irritates and worries me. I look forward to dance therapy because I like to be busy. I like to be physically active. I like music. I like to have fun with people. But I never do, really. I wind up feeling alone. I want to learn to have fun.

"It's the sexiest therapy we have. I like the pelvis stuff."

"It makes me smell. It makes me smell like a skunk. Thanks for asking."

"It is expressive and honest, and Helene is positive and pure. I was negative at first because of the name dance therapy and my own suspicion level. However, I found it to be as helpful as a session with my regular therapist. I think all patients should interact with

one another and be helpful to all. Love is essential."
Did you get anything special or unusual from dance therapy today?

"It gave me my father."

"Today, I wanted to die."

"There was some good music. There was some good dancing. There was some good walking . . .and marching. I liked the marching."

"It stimulated my brain to a higher peak . . .like an expression of love for a girl, like a blossoming rose, or a particular type of wanting. . . ."

"Dance was OK today except for the slow songs. I don't dig moving my arms around like a bird."

"My stomach feels better. I've had cramps every day for about a week. I think I'm dying or something. Next week I would like to learn a little bit about the basics of dancing. In other words, I've never taken any lessons. I just move the way I feel like when I dance, and I would like to be shown *how* to do it so it looks good."

"All my fingers feel good."

"I learned how to move my feet forward and back."
What do you think about the circle formation that we use at the beginning of every session?

"Circles are just a symbol, with no beginning, no end . . .linking the yes/no together."

"Here is the circle as we begin—O. Here is the circle when some patients leave—o. Here it is when *you* leave——."

"Circle dancing is difficult with people working deliberately against you. I also don't like it since I can't move freely with the music. I think I do better by myself."

"I like to see the people in a circle touching hands."

"Circle moving is very good. It is a feeling of home. The people I love. My parents, my sister, my brother, my niece and nephew, and my child. My husband."

[This patient has no child, no husband, and has set her parents' bed afire.]

"A circle means security or murder. It means a psychiatrist. A pacifist. It means child slaughter."

"I don't like to trust anyone with my hand."

What kind of music do you like best?

"Very relaxing."

"I prefer rock and roll music because it turns me on. . . . it has an essential beat like my insides . . . like my blood."

"I like music . . . classical, popular, folk, spiritual, country."

"Music that makes you touch one another . . . like folk, or good jazz."

"Quiet music for the Christmas freak-out . . . or any time of year."

"Rock, rock, rock around the clock."

"The kind that makes me feel like I got balls, man, balls."

"Drums and African stuff. It really turns me on. I get really lost with drums."

Where would you rather be instead of attending a dance therapy session?

"I'd rather be with my mother on my way home to see my sister."

"Visiting my father."

"Fucking."

"I'd rather be having a baby. Is it hard to do that?"
[Written by a thirty-two-year-old woman who has no children.]

"The outside world is full of dancers and dancing. This room is like the world. But I'd rather be out there."

"I'd like to be out cutting the roses in my backyard. If someone falls on my scissors' blade . . .it can't be my fault, can it?"

"I'd like to be inventing something. A mother and a father, maybe."

"I would like to go to the movies in Philadelphia. Thank you."

"Sometimes I don't understand what you want of us."

Did the African music we heard today make you think of any animal?

"Humpback creatures and lezzies (lesbians) who come on strong in New York."

"A boa constrictor to squeeze the life out of you. You're such a snot."

"I thought of a monkey, and a little girl with a lollypop. Her grandma took her to the zoo, and there was this big, ugly monkey in a cage. It pulled the little girl in and ate her up. That was a dream I had, and my therapist said I was the little girl and the monkey was my father. He's right."

I have also received unsolicited letters from patients and therapists, which are pinned up on the office bulletin board, waiting for me when I come to work.

One day I found an envelope tacked up on the bulletin board and addressed to "Crazy Helene." It had been carefully sealed with cellophane tape. When I opened it, there was a letter and a freshly pressed man's handkerchief, enclosed as a gift. The letter read:

Dear Helene,

If you want to get married to me, here's how you do it. First of all don't mention it to anybody. Secondly, tango with me forever. Thirdly, see to it that I change with the seasons. For I am sick. Dammit!

Love,
Jack

Jack, twenty-four years old, had written the letter after he had attended several dance therapy sessions. He had consistently refused to work with the group, but had elected to dance solely with me, in an exaggerated tango movement. Each time his leg restraints had been removed at my request, and it became my responsibility to see that he didn't run out the door and disappear over the hills as was his custom if unattended. Although he had never said a word to me or to anyone else in the room, I made a point of being extremely talkative with him. I began each session by explaining to him my responsibility for him, my trust in him, my expectations of him. His response each time was to put out his arms to me, hold me in a close embrace, and tango for the first five minutes of the session. For that period of time, there was no music in the room, just the sound of his labored, shallow breathing, and in tango rhythm, his humming. He watched the group from the sidelines after that, seemingly content, his blue eyes twinkling, his face a smiling Buddha, as if some inscrutable secret were locked in his person. But not once did he glance at the door marked "Exit."

Jack's letter reminded me that while a dance therapist is primarily concerned with nonverbal communication, sometimes the verbal or written message goes straight to the mark. Any tool that gives the therapist additional insights is worthy of inclusion in her mixed bag of approaches, and the written responses I received from my patients provided me with rich material for further sessions.

For example, I was able to structure our time to meet a specific need from information I gleaned from Don's answer to what he would rather be doing instead of dance therapy: "I'd rather be with my mother on my way home to see my sister." Knowing in advance of the love-hate dependency Don had for his mother, knowing too that he had only a brother with whom he was highly competitive, Don's answer was loaded with the dynamics of his case. I decided to make it possible for Don to create a scene based on the emotions that he had inadvertently exposed in answering my question.

Since we were approaching the Christmas season, it seemed natural to play "Jingle Bells" on the record player. Soon, light, tinkling sounds of music pervaded the room, sounds made for childlike skipping and walking and prancing. It was irresistible, and the group was quickly involved in a prance that duplicated the movements of three-year-old children.

125

"Don," I said, "how about a walk with your mother?" Watching an expression of surprise slowly encompass Don's face, I added, "You wrote that you'd rather be taking a walk with your mother on the way home to see your sister instead of coming to dance therapy. Do you remember writing that?"

Don shook his head. "Nope, but I'll do it, anyhow. It sounds like it'd be OK."

"May I be your mother?" Brian said in a simpering, exaggeratedly feminine manner.

Don looked at him intensely for a moment. "OK, you'll do." He looked carefully around the room. "And for my sister —I want Penny."

Penny clapped her hands and jumped up and down like a kid at a party. "Goody goody, I'm the baby sister."

Brian linked his arm through Don's. "Let's go for a walk, sonny," he said.

"C'mon, gang," I called to the rest of the patients. "We're all going for a walk with Don and his mother, on our way to visit his sister."

Don now warmed to the plan. "C'mon mommy, step carefully. There are holes in the snow and you might fall through." Brian and Don walked carefully around the room lifting their feet to avoid the danger spots that Don had discovered.

"Where are we going, Don?" I asked.

"To my sister's," Don answered. He cupped his hand over his mouth, and in a stage whisper continued, "Mom doesn't know this, but she's going to fall down in the snow soon. It's going to be very cold, and she's going to freeze."

"Will you help her up out of the snow?" I asked.

126

"Nope," he said matter of factly. "We've had a nice walk, but now it's over. I'm going to leave her in the snow ...to freeze to death."

As we all gamboled around mother and son to the continuing lilt of "Jingle Bells," Brian suddenly slid to the floor, no doubt prodded by an elbow from Don. He looked somewhat startled as he lay there.

"Oooh," Carol said, "looks like mommy's on her can!"

Brian looked up plaintively. "Help me up, son," he squealed. "It's cold down here."

Don looked down for a moment, his face hard. "I'm splitting, Ma."

Suddenly Penny was beside him. "C'mon brother, I'm waiting for you at our house. I'm fixing Christmas dinner. Bring your friends, too." Penny waved at us all, and while mommy called and pleaded from her snowy berth, everyone gaily skipped away, in time to the music.

From Don's answer to my question had come his dance therapy Christmas present—a happy farewell to his dominating mother, and a lovely transfer of an annoying brother to a charming sister.

Then there was Carol's answer to my question of "Did the African music we heard today make you think of any animal?": "Humpback creatures and lezzies (lesbians) who come on strong in New York." Through staff meetings, I became aware that Carol had some strong homosexual leanings, and that an experience with a roommate in New York had left her with unresolved guilt feelings. Could I create a "New York scene" that would make her experience seem so universal as to be unthreatening? Or, failing that, using dance therapy, could I expose Carol to the intense quality of friendship which is possible between women, and which is devoid of sexual overtones?

For my mood music, I decided to use the score from "Midnight Cowboy," a searing musical commentary on the loneliness and depravity of every big city.

"Carol, let's do a scene from your life in New York, you know, some of the scary types that you wrote me about—misshapen creatures and 'lezzies' coming at you from all directions."

Carol had been slumped in a corner and now she raised her head in dismay. "Oh, Christ, if I have to dance, I will. But that stuff is too heavy. Can't we just dance?"

"Well, this is dance, too," I said. "It's just working two things together, a lot of body and some head work with it."

"Hey," Penny asked, "how do you know which to trust, Mrs. L.? My body can make it on its own, but man, my mind is really screwed up!"

"You know what my therapist says?" Laura answered for me. "If you don't block either one with crap, you can trust 'em both."

I patted Carol on the head. "Just play it low key. Let it happen naturally."

At that, Penny hunched her shoulders, stuck her tongue in her cheek, and became an instant Quasimodo. "C'mon, Carol, I tripped once in Sin City, I know the types. Let's do it."

Carol looked up at the grimacing Penny. "Outa sight!" she said. "OK, here I come!" Carol raised her shoulders up to her ears, screwed her face into a grotesque, one-eyed mask, bowed her legs, made claws of her fingers, and descended menacingly upon Laura. Laura, genuinely frightened, made a small monkey face, squealed, and began backing up fearfully.

128

Pencil and Paper Approaches

Penny leaped in front of Laura. "Stop picking on innocent young girls, you dirty lez. I'm your type. Try me," she cackled.

The two girls—menacing ogres—faced each other. Now their finger-claws were interlaced, and their bodies rocked from side to side. They crossed their eyes, they spit at one another, but their bodies seemed stalled in neutral gear. Suddenly, with a shriek from Carol, they let loose, and wrestled one another to the floor. At first, Carol's long arms seemed to pin Penny down, but then in an instant, wiry, spunky Penny was on top. For a second their eyes met, and Penny giggled, all the fight out of her body. Then both girls relaxed in each others arms, laughing and rocking and hugging one another.

"You are some crazy lezzie," Carol laughed. "Why did you look so ugly? What the fuck did you want from me anyways?"

"Ah, that was just to scare you. You know, like I was a big-city type. I'm just a good kid like you ... stuck in shitty city. Wanna be friends?"

"Yeah," Carol said softly, "let's be buddies." The girls helped each other up, and then walked off the floor together with the strains of "Midnight Cowboy" swelling up on cue. They were holding hands very naturally, something neither of them would have dared to do an hour before, nor would I have thought of initiating the setting if I had not read Carol's revealing answer.

However, letters from patients are not the only sources of inspiration for a session. There are times when a letter from another dance therapist, or a budding therapist, whose perspective is far enough away to be objective, can reaffirm the purpose of the sessions.

I received such a letter recently. It was from a young lady who, though both a dancer and a teacher, was so impressed

129

with our sessions, that she decided to take her graduate work in dance therapy and enter the field as a qualified professional. She wrote:

Dear Helene,

Watching your work and talking with you confirmed my desire to become a dance therapist. The picture I saw in the recreation room—everyone cradling and rocking each other in their arms on that day when violent vibrations had made everyone afraid and hostile—will remain with me for a long time.

Sincerely,
Irene

Epilogue

What *is* the power of dance?

Deep in the forest primeval, hands clasped, eyes turned toward one another, our ancestors the chimps hooted and stomped from one leg to another. They danced out of fear, out of anxiety, out of the sheer ecstasy of triumph in combat.

Aeons later, early man danced. With lightning playing around his cave, he wandered out, mesmerized, propelled by a drive to commune with the unknown. His body whipped, bent, pushed, explored, as he danced his challenge to the all-powerful elements. Cowering together in the darkness of the cave, the timid ones gaped, awestruck by his audacity. Moved by what they saw, a slight figure with arms outstretched, weaving against the horizon, others painted his picture on the walls of the cave.

Today, we employ the power of dance in a new setting. The cowering figures of the cave are now members of an "advanced" society, many of whom lack any sense of their bodily needs. To these frozen, wordless, rejected humans, the dance therapist addresses herself.

Because mental health depends in part upon the body's muscular ability to stay flexible and pliable, the dance therapist must first evaluate the areas of rigidity in her patients. Why does a man hold his head stiffly apart from his body? Can he not bear to be associated with it? Whom does the clenched fist want to punch? If the young girl relaxes her tight mouth, will she say words that are too painful to hear? Why does one patient rigidly contract his pelvis? Is he afraid of proclaiming his manhood? Does the young boy keep his arms pinned to his sides because he might strangle his mother—or hug her? When the red-haired woman speaks in jumbled sentence patterns, what is she trying *not* to say?

The dance therapist observes also that some of her patients are obese from overeating, some skeleton-thin from willful starvation, some bald from frenzied plucking. She muses on the desperation that has made a man's fingers claw layers of skin from his face.

Myriad questions puzzle the dance therapist, who is not a psychiatrist, and who is certainly not a witch doctor. She is a person who has learned through her reading, training, and practice that a body with tensely locked musculature can only make incomplete, clonic movements. These movements cannot send clear signals to the brain since the synapses which pass on nervous impulses remain closed. Only the complete tonic movements of a healthy, aligned body can promote a free system of communication between body and brain. The dance therapist works at making a patient's gestures and movements strong, meaningful, larger than life, in order to open the "locked" synapses.

In a dance therapy session the patient has an opportunity to enlarge his physical vocabulary, to stretch and use his muscles, and to rediscover forgotten parts of his body. He also has the chance to be with others in a social situation, which if handled well by the therapist, can provide him with an unthreatening, good-humored environment in which to develop.

Marian Chace, the dance therapist *extraordinaire*, has written: "The question is often asked as to whether dancing is a cure. This is not the function of dance therapy. It is one of the ways in which people who are mentally ill can be with one another without too much fear of defeat. This, in itself, is relaxing, quite aside from the effects of body exercise. It is one of the ways in which patients can again begin to feel themselves a definite part of a group of people, and begin, in a small way, to function again in society." (Marian Chace, "Opening Doors Through Dance," *Journal of the American Association for Health, Physical Education and Recreation,* Vol. 23, [March, 1952]: p. 10, 11+.)

When I began my training at Philadelphia State Hospital, there was no fully developed academic program for dance therapists. Consequently, dancers were forced to develop their own methods and techniques, resulting in standards that were not uniform. Today, a growing number of educational facilities offer "field of interest" courses to dance majors, as well as degrees in dance therapy at the graduate and undergraduate levels. Two schools which offer programs that have gained national recognition are Hunter College in New York City, which offers a master's program in dance therapy, and Texas Institute of Child Psychiatry at Texas Children's Hospital, Houston, Texas, which offers a training course leading to certification in dance therapy.

In 1966, I received my initial training in dance therapy from Beth Kalish, a dedicated woman and highly skilled professional, who was then the dance therapist at Philadelphia State Hospital. Largely through her efforts, the emergence of the American Dance Therapy Association (ADTA) took place, giving cohesion and structure to struggling dance therapists throughout the country. Since its inception in 1966, ADTA has grown and developed and is currently interrelated with the disciplines of psychology, psychiatry, anthropology, and education. New insights into human development and health have been gained by this interchange of ideas between the professions.

The ADTA holds one general conference annually in various parts of the country, and weekend seminars and workshops take place throughout the year. A newsletter is sent to members four times a year, as well as a copy of the bylaws, the code of ethics, and a membership list.

The ADTA keeps its members informed of educational programs as they are instituted around the country. For the established dance therapist, the ADTA provides a registry of dance therapists. Registry listing is based on education and experience in the field. The registry's criteria serve as guidelines for prospective dance therapists, employing institutions, and the structuring of college curricula. The association also maintains bibliographies of books and journal articles, as well as unpublished manuscripts and films. Information can be obtained by writing to the American Dance Therapy Association, 10400 Connecticut Avenue, Suite 300, Kensington, Maryland 20795.

Founded in 1940, the Dance Notation Bureau Center for Movement Research and Analysis is another center for dance therapy information and education. Through its school and library, the Bureau augments the understanding of human movement. The teaching of Rudolph Laban's two systems, "Labananalysis" and "Effort/Shape," comprise the core of the school's program. Fundamental to both systems is the recording and analysis of the process of an action, which preserves the exact pattern of any kind of physical action and creates a score similar to that used by musicians. Effort/Shape analysis has found its place in areas that study expressive and behavioral aspects of movement. The dance therapist may use it in recording patterns of movement as an aid in personality assessment.

Courses, training programs, and bibliography in the growing field of dance therapy are provided by the Dance Notation Bureau. Information on membership can be obtained from the Dance Notation Bureau, 19 Union Square West, New York, New York 10003.

Appendix A
Suggested Reading List

The following is my personal reading list and includes books that have been helpful, informative, and stimulating to me.

Ardrey, Robert. *African Genesis*. New York: Atheneum, 1961.

Bartenieff, Irmgard, and Davis, Martha. "Effort/Shape Analysis of Movement. Unity of Expression and Function." Manuscript available, Dance Notation Bureau, New York City, 1965.

Birdwhistle, Ray L.—Any of his articles.

Buckle, Richard. *Nijinsky*. New York: Simon and Schuster, 1971.

Chace, Marian.—Any of her articles.

Duncan, Isadora. *The Art of Dance*. New York: Theatre Art Books, 1969.

Erikson, Erik H. *Childhood and Society.* New York: W.Ẇ. Norton and Co., Inc., 1950.

Faraday, Anne. *Dream Power.* New York: Coward, McCann and Geoghegan, 1972.

Fenichel, Otto. *Psychiatry of Neurosis.* New York: W. W. Norton and Co., Inc., 1945.

Grotowski, Jerzy. *Towards a Poor Theatre.* New York: Simon and Schuster, 1968.

Harris, Thomas A. *I'm O.K., You're O.K.* New York: Harper & Row, 1969.

Haskell, Arnold. *The Wonderful World of Dance.* Garden City: Doubleday and Co., Inc., 1970.

Holt, John. *Freedom and Beyond.* New York: E. P. Dutton and Co., 1973.

Honig, Albert. *The Awakening Nightmare*, Rockaway, New Jersey: American Faculty Press, 1972.

Humphrey, Doris. *The Art of Making Dances.* New York: Grove Press, 1959.

Janov, Arthur. *The Primal Scream.* New York: G. B. Putnam Sons, 1970.

———. *The Anatomy of Mental Illness.* New York: G. B. Putnam Sons, 1971.

Laing, R. D. *The Divided Self.* Baltimore: Penguin Books, 1965.

Lowen, Alexander. *The Behavior of the Body.* New York: McMillan and Co., 1967.

Maslow, Abraham.—Any of his books.

Perls, Frederick. *Gestalt Therapy: Excitement and Growth in Human Personality.* New York: Dell Books, 1965.

Pesso, Albert. *Movement in Psychotherapy: Psychomotor Techniques and Training.* New York University Press, 1969.

Sachs, Curt. *World History of Dance.* New York: W. W. Norton and Co., Inc., 1937.

Schilder, Paul. *The Image and Appearance of the Human Body.* New York: International University Press, 1970.

Stebbins, G. *Delsarte: System of Expression.* London: Werner, 1887.

Spolen, Viola. *Improvisations for the Theatre.* Chicago: Northwestern University Press, 1963.

Woolf, Virginia. *To the Lighthouse.* New York: Modern Library, 1937.

————.*Mrs. Dalloway.* Middlesex, England: Penguin Books, 1964.

Appendix B
Suggested Record List

For me, there is nothing like music for inspiring the human body to move, to run, to leap with joy. Because I am stirred by music, it would be unthinkable for me to have a dance therapy session without the stimulus of music. Although some of my colleagues feel that they can attain good results by substituting mechanical aids, e.g. ropes, rubber bands, balls, scarves, etc., which initiate movement, in my view, *music* is the prime stimulant to movement.

For dance therapy purposes, I have one requisite: the music must have a steady, strong beat for if the beat is not strong and forceful, the patient's attention will wander. Just as my enthusiasm and zest must inspire a patient to get off his chair and onto his feet, so must the music dynamically inspire him. When my mood is reflective and uncertain, the patients, sensing my lack of direction, go adrift with me. To be effective

141

in a dance therapy session, music must have the power to quicken pulses, to strike sparks in the decaying spirit of the patient.

Although the list of recordings that follows is short, it indicates the kind of music that my patients requested over and over. Since trends in music change, however, and young patients most often follow the trends, the dance therapist will want to keep her list current.

To this end, I recommend the following:

BB King	Indianola Mississippi Seeds	ABC Dunhill Records, Inc.
Traffic	High Heeled Boys	Island Artists
Hugh Masekela	The Promise of a Future	Universal City Records
The Karmon Israeli Folk Dancers and Singers	Song of the Sabras	Vanguard
The Best of Wilson Pickett	Volume 11	Atlantic Recording D.
Elton John	Honky Chateau	Strawberry Studios, France
John Williams	Two Guitar Concertos	Columbia Masterworks
Igor Stravinsky	Firebird Suite	Music Appreciation Records
Brahms	Eight Hungarian Dances	Columbia Masterworks

Appendix

James Taylor	Sweet Baby James	Warner Brothers Records
Stan Getz	Didn't We	Ja Ma Music Co.
Carole King	Tapestry	Columbia Music, Inc.
Blood, Sweat, and Tears	Volume 2	Columbia Records
Johnny Menko	Polkas	Fiesta Records
The United States Marine Band	Album of Marches	Radio Corporation of America
Dizzy Gillespie	Echoes of an Era	Roulette
Ginger Baker	Fela Ransome-Kuti and the Africa '70	Signpost Records
Janis Joplin	Pearl	Columbia Records
Olatunji	Flaming Drums	Columbia Records
Laurindo Almeida	The Guitar Worlds of Laurindo Almeida	Capitol
Modern Jazz Quartet	One Never Knows	Atlantic Recording
Dvorák	New World Symphony	RCA Victor
Ravel	Boléro-Rapsodie Espagnole	Command Classics

About the author

Helene Lefco has always danced. She says, "From the age of three when I thumped my bottom to the beat of the Charleston to today when I unselectively dance to Vivaldi as well as rock . . . I have danced."

She has formally studied the disciplines of Martha Graham, Hanya Holm, Weidman, Humphrey, Mary Wigman, and Limón. Her early training in dance therapy was done with therapists in New York, Pennsylvania, and Washington, D.C., the most important influence being a series of training sessions with the pioneer dance therapist, Marion Chace, of St. Elizabeth's Hospital in Washington.

Of Marion Chace, Mrs. Lefco says, "This lady's influence upon me, both personally and professionally, has been profound. A truly sensitive and intuitive woman, who came to each session with astounding freshness and flexibility, (she) taught me by example that a dance therapist's greatest asset is her instinctive joy of movement. It is this primal spontaneity which should be transmitted to one's patients."

After graduating from New York University with a degree in communications, she was a feature writer for *Vogue*, a publicist for Paramount Pictures, and a freelance writer for the *Ladies Home Journal*, the *Philadelphia Bulletin*, the *Philadelphia Inquirer*, and other publications. She is married and the mother of three children.

As a dance therapist she has worked in a state hospital with regressed, tranquilized cases, in a private clinic with unmedicated patients, and currently she is dance therapist at Delaware Valley Mental Health Foundation at Doylestown, Pennsylvania.